Cancer of the Larynx and Hypopharynx

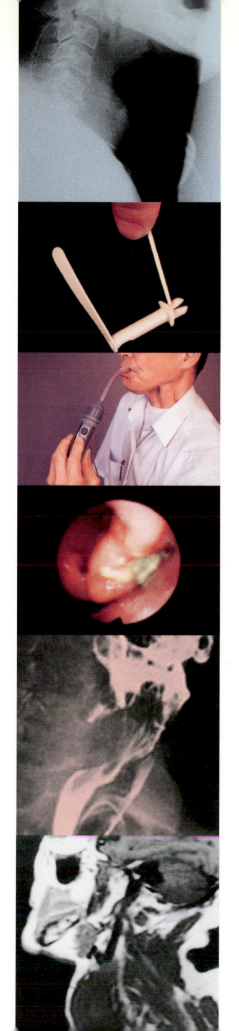

Cancer of the Larynx and Hypopharynx

By

William I. Wei MBBS MS FRCS(ENG)
FRCS(EDIN) FACS FHKAM(SURG) FHKAM(ORL)
*W. Mong Chair of Otorhinolaryngology
and Professor of Surgery,
The University of Hong Kong,
Queen Mary Hospital, Hong Kong*

and

Jonathan S.T. Sham MD FRCR DMRT FHKCR
*Professor, Department of Clinical Oncology,
The University of Hong Kong,
Queen Mary Hospital, Hong Kong*

I S I S
MEDICAL
MEDIA

© 2000 by Isis Medical Media Ltd.
59 St. Aldates
Oxford OX1 1ST, UK

First published 2000

British Library Cataloguing in Publication Data.
A catalogue record for this title is available from
the British Library

ISBN 1 899066 64 0

Wei, W.I. (William)
Cancer of the Larynx and Hypopharynx
William I. Wei, Jonathan S.T. Sham

Always refer to the manufacturer's Prescribing
Information before prescribing drugs cited in this book.

Typsetting and image reproduction by
Color Gallery Sdn Bhd, Malaysia

Artwork by
Anna Maria Dutto

Isis Medical Media staff
Commissioning Editor: Jonathan Gregory
Editorial Controller: Fiona Cornell
Production Managers: Julia Savory, Sarah Sodhi

Printed and bound by
Craft Print Pte Ltd., Singapore

Distributed in the USA by
Books International Inc., P.O. Box 605,
Herndon, VA 20172, USA

Distributed in the rest of the world by
Plymbridge Distributors Ltd., Estover Road,
Plymouth, PL6 7PY, UK

contents

Squamous cell carcicoma of the larynx and hypopharynx is a lifestyle disease caused virtually always by smoking cigarettes and drinking alcohol, usually in prodigious quantities. Most of these cancers present in advanced stages of the disease. Despite the introduction of various chemotherapeutic agents and improvement in radiation therapy, surgery remains the basic approach to these problems.

This book, *Cancer of the Larynx and Hypopharynx*, is a book by surgeons for surgeons. The details of diagnosis, surgical management, reconstruction, and rehabilitation described herein are based upon the extensive experience of the authors' contributions to the scientific literature on this topic. Conservation surgery as well as considerable details on pre-and postoperative care and reconstruction is provided. Appropriately, little emphasis is placed on treatment by chemotherapy and/or radiation, even in advanced stage disease.

The book is excellent, richly illustrated and makes extensive use of the boxes and algorithms to summarize salient points in management which would also make this valuabe for students and early residents. This book, which is compact and concisely written, has much to offer to those interested in the management of cancer of the larynx and hypopharynx. Professor Wei is to be congratulated on the leadership he has provided in the advances in the management of this disease and his dedication to sharing his experience and contributions with us.

Eugene N. Myers, M.D.
Professor and Chairman,
Department of Otolaryngology,
University of Pittsburgh School of Medicine,
Pittsburgh, Pennsylvania, USA

Management of cancer in the laryngeal and hypopharyngeal regions remains a challenge. The location of the cancer makes precise determination of the extent of the malignancies difficult. Frequently, patients are not in optimal clinical condition and the decision has to be made for the selection of the appropriate therapeutic measure. Treatment of these neoplasms may disturb their speech and swallowing abilities. When patients present in advanced stages of the disease, combined modality of therapy may have to be instituted.

The book aims to address all these problems within 150 pages and is written for the young otorhinolaryngologists, head and neck surgeons, clinical oncologists and rehabilitation personnel. The chapters are arranged in two sections. The section on cancer of the larynx starts with the diagnostic procedures and the range of therapeutic options. Subsequent focus is on results of current treatment modalities and procedures of voice rehabilitation. The management of the cervical lymph nodes, an integral part of treatment is also included. The section on cancer of the hypopharynx has emphasis on the therapeutic aspect. The concept of adequate resection followed by appropriate reconstruction is presented and the importance of combined treatment modality is stressed. Complications and their management following therapies are important and two separate chapters are devoted to it.

The authors are practicing otorhinolaryngologists, head and neck surgeons and clinical oncologists. The latter has contributed chapters 5 and 12, while the former has contributed the other chapters. Clinical photographs together with line drawings illustrating the practical aspect of patient management form a salient part of the book. Algorithms and boxes containing key issues are frequently used throughout the chapters; through these the reader will appreciate the crucial points more readily.

It is our hope that this book will be a useful tool to physicians interested in the pathology, diagnosis, treatment and rehabilitation of patients suffering from cancer of the larynx and hypopharynx.

W.I. Wei
J.S.T. Sham

Acknowledgement

We are greatly indebted to Professor G.B. Ong, John H.C. Ho, John Wong and K.H. Lam, from whom we have acquired clinical experience and knowledge; to students and residents from whom we have gathered enthusiasm; and to our patients from whom we have gained the drive to seek solutions for diseases.

W.I. Wei
J.S.T. Sham

To our families, whose devotion, understanding and tolerance have allowed us to contribute towards academic medicine.

W.I. Wei
J.S.T. Sham

CANCER OF THE LARYNX

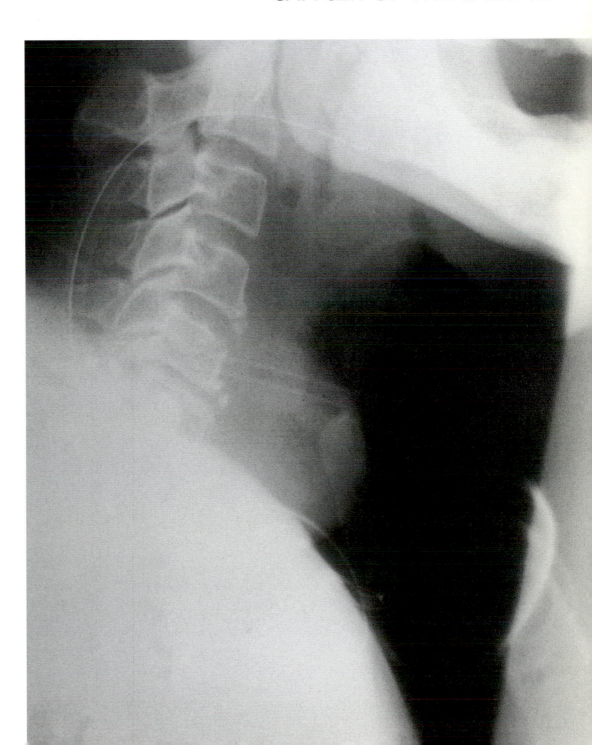

CHAPTER one

Evaluation of extent
of laryngeal cancer

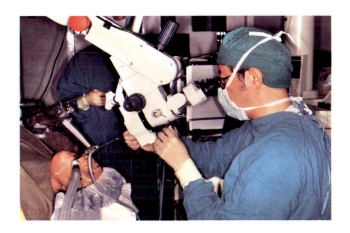

Symptomatology

Symptoms of carcinoma of the larynx are related to the size and location of the lesion within the larynx.

For carcinomas arising from the supraglottic larynx, throat discomfort, irritation and cough are early symptoms of tumour. When tumours increase in size or begin to ulcerate, haemoptysis or disturbances of swallowing may take place. With a tumour located at the laryngeal surface of the epiglottis leading to partial obstruction of the laryngeal inlet, the patient may present with inspiratory stridor (Fig. 1.1).

Hoarseness is invariably the early symptom of carcinoma situated at the glottic larynx. The presence of a growth over the vocal cords (Fig. 1.2) affects their approximation for voice production. With tumour growth and ulceration, the patient may experience haemoptysis or even airway obstruction.

Tumour in the subglottic region usually presents at an advanced stage because small tumours in the region have only trivial effects, and the patient may remain asymptomatic. When the tumour extends upwards to affect the vocal cords directly, the patient will have hoarseness. Circumferential growth may present with increasing stridor when the tumour bulk reduces the size of the airway.

When the tumour metastasizes to the cervical lymph nodes, a situation which is particularly common in the supraglottic carcinoma, the patient will present with metastatic enlargement of neck nodes, the locations being most frequently in levels II, III and IV (Fig. 1.3) (Table 1.1).

Clinical assessment

Clinical assessment of carcinoma of the larynx starts with percutaneous palpation of the laryngeal skeleton. Advanced stage laryngeal carcinoma may cause expansion of the whole cartilaginous framework and, in some patients, the tumour may even infiltrate the overlying skin (Fig. 1.4), although this is not usual. Both sides of the neck should be palpated for enlarged cervical lymph nodes

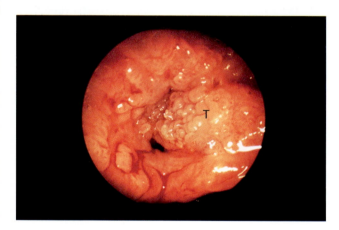

Figure 1.1 Endoscopic view of a carcinoma of the larynx (T) causing near-complete obstruction of the laryngeal inlet. This patient presents with inspiratory stridor.

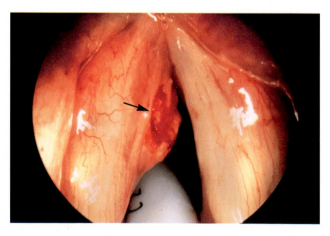

Figure 1.2 A small tumour over the anterior part of the vocal cord (arrow), impairing the approximation of the cords, leading to hoarseness.

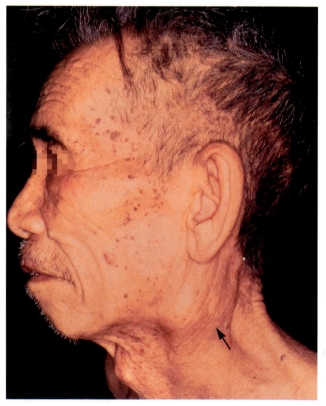

Figure 1.3 Clinical photograph of a patient suffering from carcinoma of the larynx and presenting with an enlarged level II cervical lymph node (arrow).

Table 1.1 *Symptoms related to the location of laryngeal cancer*

Location of primary tumour	Early disease	Advanced disease
Supraglottic	Disturbance of swallowing	Hoarseness, dysphagia
Glottic	Hoarseness	Airway obstruction
Subglottic	Mild haemoptysis	Hoarseness, airway obstruction

and any suspicious node, especially located in levels II, III and IV, may require further investigation.

Examination of the larynx, indirectly, with a mirror should be carried out in the clinic under local anaesthesia. If the patient can happily tolerate the mirror examination, then even spraying of the posterior pharyngeal wall with lignocaine can be omitted. Indirect examination of the larynx with the mirror allows visualization of the epiglottis and the supraglottic region. In some cooperative patients, the vocal cords can be seen in their entirety, although under most circumstances only the mobility of the vocal cords can be ascertained. However, with use of the mirror, visualization of the laryngeal surface of the epiglottis, the anterior commissure and the subglottic regions is difficult. Nevertheless, as indirect examination of the larynx using a mirror is a simple, non-invasive procedure, a large amount of information may be gathered; consequently, this should be the first procedure performed in patients suspected of suffering from carcinoma of the larynx.

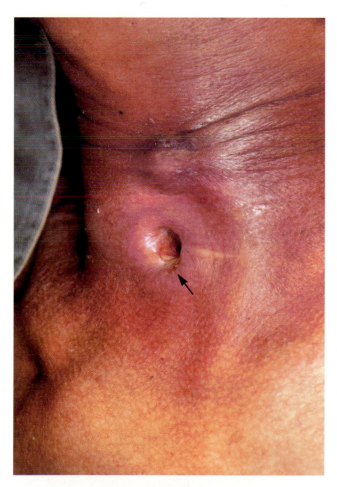

Figure 1.4 Clinical photograph of the neck of a patient suffering from carcinoma of the larynx which has extended to the anterior neck skin. This advanced tumour has also led to a compromised airway; thus, a tracheostomy was performed to relieve the obstruction (arrow).

Endoscopic assessment

With the current developments of endoscopes and their application in laryngology, it is possible to achieve a detailed examination of the larynx. Endoscopic examination using either flexible endoscopes or rigid Hopkin's rods can be carried out under local anaesthesia. In this way, a thorough examination of the larynx can be made. When the examination is performed under general anaesthesia, the operating microscope can be used to obtain a detailed examination of the different regions of the larynx under magnification. A rigid Hopkin's rod can be employed by applying it close to any macroscopic suspicious areas; this constitutes 'contact laryngoscopy'.

Flexible endoscopy

In those patients who are unable to tolerate the laryngeal mirror examination, the larynx can be adequately inspected with the aid of a flexible endoscope. This procedure can be performed under local anaesthesia with minimal disturbance of the patient. A flexible bronchoscope with a suction channel is preferred as the removal of mucus is essential to obtain an unobstructed view of the larynx. The suction channel also allows the passing of biopsy forceps to the suspicious area in order to obtain tissue for histological examination.

The flexible endoscope has the further advantage that, when it is manipulated beyond the vocal cords, an adequate vision of the subglottic region can be achieved. The entire examination is performed under local anaesthesia (Fig. 1.5). The patient is requested to vocalize while the examiner looks at the vocal cords, thus allowing the mobility of the cords to be ascertained. The nearby hypopharynx and cervical oesophagus can also be examined when the endoscope is passed once [1] (Figs 1.6, 1.7).

As the patient is fully awake during the whole procedure, they will not aspirate the small amount of bleeding that may accompany biopsy of the larynx, thus adding to the safety of the procedure.

Rigid endoscopy

Although the flexible endoscope can achieve a direct view of the laryngeal inlet and is associated with minimal morbidity, it is nevertheless an invasive procedure.

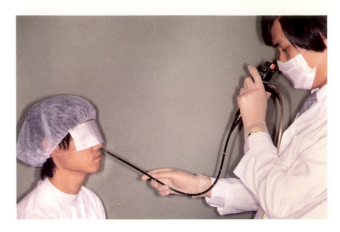

Figure 1.5 The patient sits in front of the examiner. The flexible tip of the endoscope is inserted into the nostril of the patient. The endoscope is then manipulated under direct vision through the nasal cavity, the nasopharynx and the oropharynx to reach the laryngopharyngeal region.

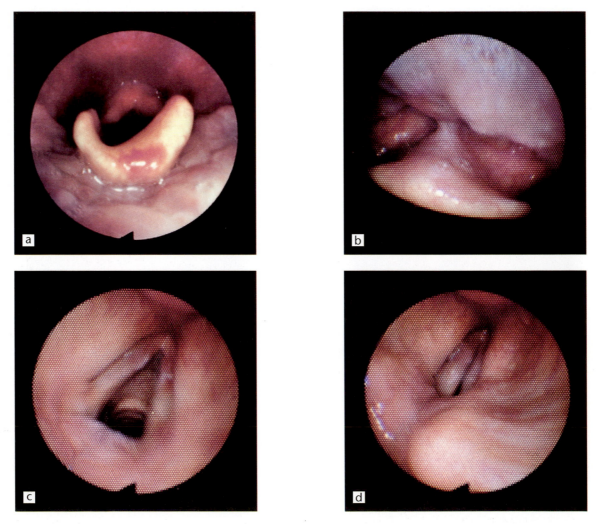

Figure 1.6 (a) Endoscopic view of the normal epiglottis. (b) The patient is requested to protrude his tongue and thus the vallecula can be adequately visualized. (c) Endoscopic view of the normal vocal cords on abduction. (d) Endoscopic view of the normal vocal cords on adduction.

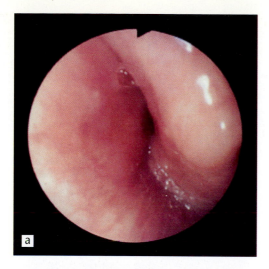
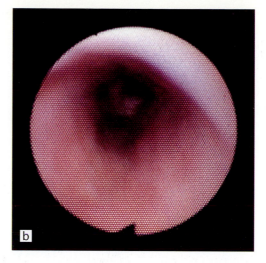

Figure 1.7 (a) Endoscopic view of the left piriform sinus. (b) Endoscopic view of the oesophagus through the fibreoptic bronchoscope. A stream of air is insufflated through the biopsy channel to distend the oesophageal mucosa.

Introduction of the endoscope through the nostril does cause some discomfort and may lead to epistaxis (Fig. 1.8). The rigid endoscope introduced transorally under local anaesthesia may also provide a good view of the laryngeal inlet (Fig. 1.9).

The images obtained from the 70° or the 90° rigid Hopkin's rods supersede those of the best flexible endo-scope. However, it is difficult to obtain a good view of the whole laryngeal inlet without the cooperation of the patient. For those patients whose vocal cords can be visualized, the mobility of the cords can be adequately documented. With the rigid endoscope, examination of the subglottic region is difficult; neither is it easy to take a biopsy of any suspicious lesion under direct vision.

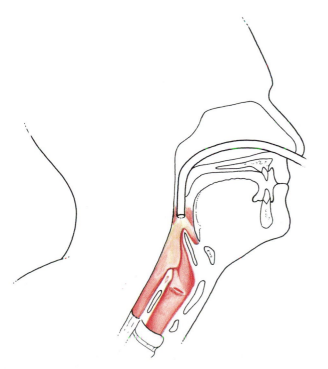

Figure 1.8 Schematic diagram to show the position of the flexible endoscope inserted through the nasal cavity, the nasopharynx and the oropharynx to reach the laryngopharyngeal region.

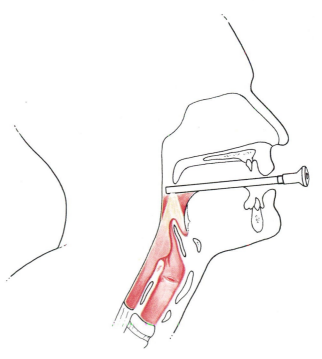

Figure 1.9 Schematic diagram to show the position of the rigid endoscope inserted through the oral cavity and oropharynx to examine the laryngopharyngeal region.

Nowadays, a camera attached to the endoscope can transfer the image onto a monitor. In this way, the entire examination can be carried out with the investigator watching the monitor screen, which avoids them straining their neck or eyes. Simultaneous photographic documentation with either a still camera or a video is also possible (Table 1.2).

Microlaryngoscopy (see Box 1.1)

Despite the technological advances in both flexible and rigid endoscopes, it is difficult in some patients to examine the larynx thoroughly under local anaesthesia. This may be due either to the patient's apprehension or to anatomical variations. This is particularly so when biopsy has to be carried out for lesions located at crucial areas, such as the anterior commissure or the subglottic region. The amount of tissue obtained for biopsy through the flexible endoscope under local anaesthesia is usually limited.

Examination of the larynx under general anaesthesia with a suspension laryngoscope and magnification through an operating microscope enables a detailed examination of the entire mucosal surface of the larynx (Fig. 1.10).

Under general anaesthesia, ventilation of the patient can be maintained through a small endotracheal tube or a 'high-frequency jet' placed at some distance above the vocal cords. The aim is to provide maximum exposure of the laryngeal inlet for examination. The laryngoscope

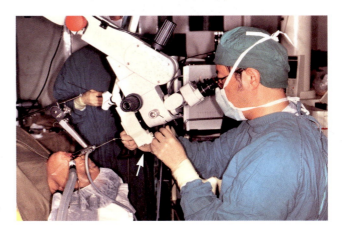

Figure 1.10 The suspension laryngoscope is inserted under general anaesthesia. The operating microscope is used for detailed examination of the larynx. Both hands of the surgeon are freed to allow use of the instruments, or to control the micromanipulator of the CO_2 laser (arrow) to perform endolaryngeal surgery.

can then be introduced to reveal the appropriate areas of the larynx and, with the accompanying suspension system, the scope can be kept in its desired position through the various anchorage attachments. This will free the surgeon's hands so that instruments passed through the laryngoscope can be used on the laryngeal structures. Rigid endoscopes can be introduced for examination – especially the 90° viewing endoscopes – and this contributes to the visualization of hidden pathologies.

The operating microscope can then be moved in to allow visualization of the various parts of the larynx under direct vision. Excess mucus in the larynx can be removed with a sucker under direct vision, and at the same time normal structures in the larynx can be retracted or manipulated to gain better exposure for detailed examination (Fig. 1.11). The examination should always include the 'paralaryngeal' area, such as the valleculae,

Table 1.2 *Comparison of the characteristics of flexible and rigid endoscopes*

Properties	Flexible endoscope	Rigid endoscope
Anaesthesia	Local anaesthesia	Local anaesthesia
Route of insertion	Transnasal	Transoral
Patient tolerance	Good	Good
Built-in suction facility	Yes	No
Biopsy channel	Yes	No
Ease of visualization of whole larynx	Good	Fair
Photographic documentation	Fair	Good

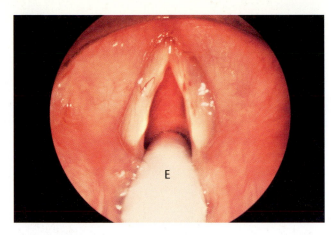

Figure 1.11 Normal vocal cords seen under magnification (×4). An endotracheal tube is used (E).

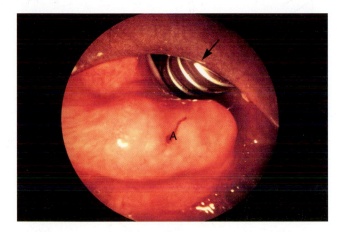

Figure 1.12 Normal left arytenoid cartilage (A) seen under magnification (×4). A metal endotracheal tube (arrow) is employed for CO_2 laser endolaryngeal surgery.

glossal surface of the epiglottis, the posterior commissure, postcricoid mucosa and the pyriform sinuses (Fig. 1.12).

The consistency or the mobility of abnormal structures in the larynx can also be tested with instruments, and biopsy of lesions at the representative area can be carried out accurately under magnification. For more extensive lesions, excisional biopsies with instruments or carbon dioxide laser can be performed with precision. When the mucosa over the whole vocal cord is thickened it can be stripped under magnification, and injury of the under-lying normal tissue is minimal.

Contact endoscopy

At the time of microlaryngoscopy, the superficial layers of the vocal cord epithelium can be examined *in vivo* and *in situ* with a rigid endoscope [2]. Methylene blue is employed initially to stain the epithelial cells of the vocal cords, and a 30° microcolpohysteroscope is applied close to the mucosa. When in contact with mucosal tissue, this endoscope allows ×60 and ×150 magnification, and the cellular pattern of the superficial cells can be visualized and documented.

A number of parameters such as the regularity of the epithelium, nucleus contour, nucleus–cytoplasm ratio and presence of mitosis can be evaluated. In-vivo observation and documentation of the vascular distribution pattern of the vocal cord mucosa is possible. Different clinical conditions such as laryngitis, dysplasia and malignancy have specific cellular patterns on contact endoscopic examination. The alterations of vascularization pattern in association with the various pathological conditions can also be recognized. The findings of contact endoscopy lead to early recognition of the clinical condition and contribute to the accuracy of performing biopsies at the appropriate area.

Stroboscopy

The light source of a stroboscope delivers light pulses at intervals of less than 0.2 second, and the sequence of pictures thus produced provides an optical illusion of continuous movement ('vibrations'). In general, the vocal cords have two movements: (i) those associated with the contraction of the muscle; and (ii) the transverse waves of the overlying mucosa. It is the changing pattern of the 'vibrations' of the mucosa that may provide a clue to an early malignancy.

The vibrations of the mucosa can be seen to be diminished when it is adherent to the underlying tissue. One of the causes is the presence of invasive carcinoma of the vocal cord. Stroboscopic examination is useful in the follow-up of patients with 'chronic laryngitis' to detect any change of mucosal wave pattern which may indicate early malignancy. Normal mucosa at the edge of the vocal cords moves up and down smoothly when examined with the stroboscope. Whenever the mucosa is tethered to any underlying structure, this gentle mucosal swinging movement will appear to be reduced or impaired. This is particularly useful in the follow-up of patients who have early carcinoma of the larynx and who have been treated with radiotherapy. Absence or reduction of the mucosal wave may indicate recurrence of tumour, and the region on the vocal cords where there is a change of wave pattern may indicate the appropriate position for biopsy.

Radiological assessments

The purpose of radiological examination is to ascertain the extent of tumour involvement and the degree of deep invasion. Conventional X-radiographic investigations such as laryngography or tomography, etc. have now been replaced by computed tomography (CT) or magnetic resonance imaging (MRI) (Table 1.3).

Computed tomography

Computed tomography can be used to demonstrate soft tissue distortion of the structures within the larynx (Fig. 1.13), and complements the endoscopic findings. This is particularly so when sections of CT are carried out at very fine intervals, when the extension of tumour to surrounding areas such as the pre-epiglottic space or the pyriform sinus can be detected. More importantly, CT can be used to demonstrate the deep invasion aspect of tumour, especially when the cartilage skeleton is invaded or destroyed by tumour (Fig. 1.14).

When the CT images include the neck region, then any lymph node metastasis which is in association with the primary carcinoma of the larynx and not palpable clinically, may be detected. Subsequent investigation such as fine needle aspiration aptology should be carried out,

and the findings of this investigation may modify the treatment plan for any particular patient.

Magnetic resonance imaging

This technique is superior to CT in its ability to better identify soft tissue. With injection of contrast, MRI can be used to differentiate tumour from its surrounding oedematous tissue, although with post-radiation tissue this differentiation is not always reliable. MRI also provides information regarding tumour invasion of the laryngeal cartilage and the lymph node status of the neck. The technique has the added advantage of obtaining the sagittal view, thus giving the impression of the vertical extent of tumour. A three-dimensional view of the laryngeal tumour can be reconstructed (Fig. 1.15). However, in those patients who have cardiac pacemakers fitted or who may have other metallic implants (e.g. mechanical heart valve), MRI should not be carried out for fear of moving these implants and CT be performed instead.

Table 1.3 *Characteristics of radiological assessments*

	Computed tomography	Magnetic resonance imaging
Assessing tumour extent	2-dimensionally	3-dimensionally
Assessing invasion of cartilage	Good	Fair
Assessing soft tissue involvement	Fair	Good
Radiation hazards	Low	Nil

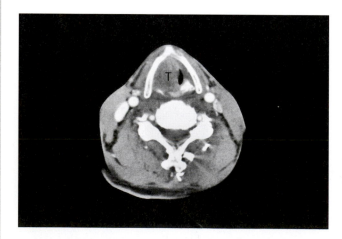

Figure 1.13 Computed tomography showing a tumour (T) causing distortion of soft tissue within the laryngeal framework.

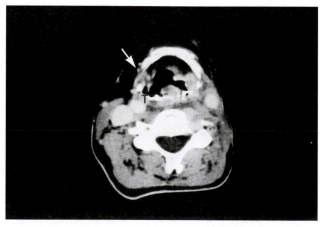

Figure 1.14 Computed tomography showing destruction of laryngeal cartilage (arrow) by laryngeal carcinoma (T).

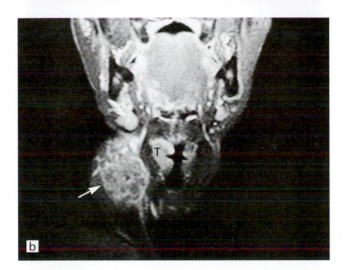

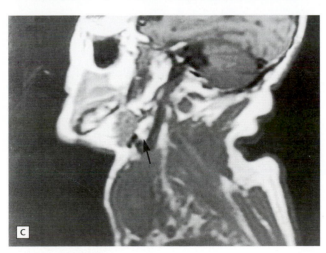

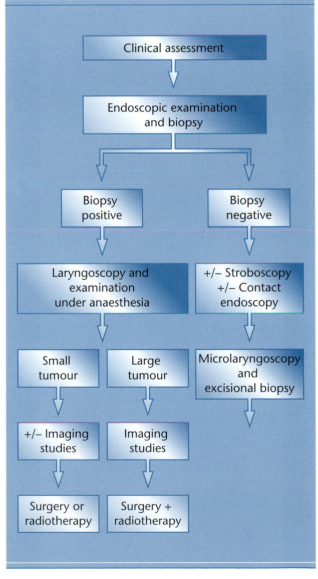

Figure 1.15 Magnetic resonance imaging showing the three-dimensional view of a laryngeal carcinoma. (a) Axial view showing tumour (T) in larynx and lymph nodes in the neck (arrow). (b) Coronal view showing tumour (T) and lymph nodes in the neck (arrow). (c) Sagittal view showing the vertical extent of tumour (arrow) in the larynx.

Summary (Fig. 1.16)

Patients suspected of suffering from carcinoma of the larynx should be examined with the laryngeal mirror and assessed clinically. A more detailed examination is possible with the use of either a flexible or rigid endoscope under local anaesthesia. The latter instrument provides a better image, but the flexible endoscope permits biopsy under direct vision. Examination under general anaesthesia with magnification allows precise determination of the extent of carcinoma over the mucosal surface. The invasion of tumour in other dimensions can be assessed with CT or MRI. Early-stage carcinoma may be detected with either stroboscopy or contact endoscopy, combined with biopsy.

Figure 1.16 Evaluation of carcinoma of the larynx.

References

1. Wei WI, Lau WF, Lam KH, Hui Y. The role of the fibreoptic bronchoscope in otorhinolaryngological practice. *J Laryngol Otol* 1987; 101: 1263–1270.

2. Andrea M, Dias O, Santos A. Contact endoscopy during microlaryngeal surgery: a new technique for endoscopic examination of the larynx. *Ann Otol Rhinol Laryngol* 1995; 104: 333–339.

CHAPTER two

Early laryngeal cancer

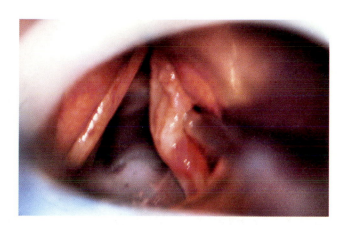

Introduction

The optimal treatment for carcinoma of the larynx is the one which will eradicate the tumour and preserve the voice while at the same time minimizing the risk of treatment for the patient (Box 2.1).

In view of management planning, the early laryngeal carcinomas mentioned here include T1, T2 and some favourable T3 glottic tumours without lymph node metastasis. These stages of tumour are considered together here, as in general the results of treatment with radiotherapy and a specific form of surgery are similar (Table 2.1). The choice between the treatment options depends on the status of the patient, the radiation facilities of the institute, and also the surgical expertise available. The patient and the family members should also be involved in the discussion of the choice of treatment method.

Radiotherapy

Supraglottic carcinoma

Radiation treatment alone for T1 tumour can achieve a disease control rate of 80–100% and for T2 tumour of 70–80% [1–3]. The local tumour control rate between the anatomical subsites within the supraglottic larynx shows no significant difference. The radiation dose delivered to the primary tumour ranges from 6000 to 6800 cGy depending on the stage, tumour volume within the stage, and the growth pattern of the tumour. In view of the relatively high incidence of metastasis to the cervical lymph nodes, the neck is included in the radiation field [4]. Radiotherapy offers the best opportunity to preserve the larynx without jeopardizing the chance of cure. Chondroradionecrosis of the laryngeal skeleton is one of the possible complications following radiotherapy, but fortunately is uncommon. The main flaw in this type of treatment is that it is difficult in an irradiated larynx to detect recurrence with clinical examination and imaging studies. As these early recurrences tend to be submucosal in location, it is difficult to obtain histological confirmation. When detected, the recurrence is usually too large for conservative surgery to be effective, and thus total laryngectomy must be carried out in order to effect salvage.

Glottic carcinoma

Carcinomas over the vocal cords are usually symptomatic because of their location. In view of the sparse lymphatic drainage of the vocal cords, carcinomas in the glottic area are usually localized in the region on presentation. The radiation dose ranges from 6000 to 7000 cGy depending on the size of the tumour and whether it has involved the anterior commissure. As these cancers rarely metastasize to the cervical lymph nodes, the irradiation field only covers the primary site, and the cervical nodes are not irradiated electively. The results of radiotherapy in controlling T1 tumour range from 85% to 95%, and for T2 tumour from 65% to 75% [5–7]. Radiotherapy is less effective when the mobility of the vocal cord decreases or when the bulky tumour extends to the subglottic area. Complications of radiotherapy such as chondroradionecrosis and laryngeal oedema are not common with the fractionation of radiation scheme currently used. Radiotherapy is an acceptable treatment option for T1 and T2 glottic cancer as the morbidity is low and voice preservation is possible. Even when tumour recurs, limited salvage surgery is frequently possible.

Box 2.1 *The aims of managing early laryngeal cancer*

- Eradicate tumour
- Preserve voice
- Cost-effective for patient

Table 2.1 *Criteria for selection of therapy for early laryngeal cancer*

	Radiotherapy	Surgery
Tumour stage	Early cancer	Early cancer
Follow-up to detect recurrence	Frequent	Regular
Complications	Chondroradionecrosis	Scar related to surgery
Problems	Difficult to detect recurrence	Lost part of larynx
Resources	Facilities and expertise	Surgical expertise

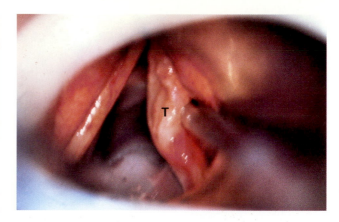

Box 2.2 *Indications for endolaryngeal surgical treatment*

- Early laryngeal carcinoma
- Facilities and surgical expertise available
- Adequate exposure of the tumour and larynx possible
- Patient agrees to further therapy if recurrence is detected

Figure 2.2 Early laryngeal carcinoma of the vocal cord which could be treated by stripping of the vocal cord mucosa (T).

Subglottic carcinoma

Early carcinoma located in the subglottic region is uncommon, as when most of these patients present with airway problems the tumour is of significant size. Radiotherapy is applicable for the few early carcinomas of the subglottic region, and a curative result has been achieved in four out of six patients [8].

Endoscopic surgery (see Box 2.2)

Microlaryngoscopic surgical resection

The success of endoscopic surgical treatment of cancer of the larynx depends on selection of the patients. Cancer of the vocal cords arises from the membranous portion of the vocal cords, the earliest cancers being carcinoma in-situ and microinvasive cancers. Pathologically, these cancers could be treated successfully with stripping of the vocal cords, thus removing the tumour. As these early cancers are frequently associated with dysplasia and hyperkeratosis of the nearby mucosa (Fig. 2.1), all the mucosae over both vocal cords – except those that constitute the anterior commissure – should be stripped to effect a curative procedure.

The procedure is performed under general anaesthesia, and ventilation of the patient may be achieved with a small endotracheal tube or high-frequency jet ventilation.

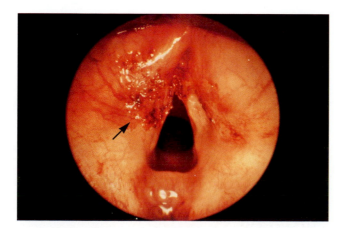

Figure 2.1 Endoscopic view of an early laryngeal carcinoma of the vocal cord with surrounding hyperkeratosis and dysplasia (arrow).

A wide-lumen laryngoscope with exposure of the anterior commissure should be used and then attached to a suspension system so that the surgeon has both hands free to carry out the surgery (Fig. 2.2). An operating microscope with a focal length of 400 mm should be used for magnification and visualization of the entire laryngeal inlet. In about 15% of patients, it is difficult to have the desired laryngoscope in position. In obese patients with a short neck and underdeveloped mandible with full dentition, it is notoriously difficult to insert a laryngoscope to expose the larynx adequately. Other patients who have cervical arthritis or stiff neck tissue following radiotherapy may not be suitable for this procedure, for similar reasons.

The free edge of the mucosa over the vocal cord is grasped with a microforceps at about 2 mm posterior to the anterior commissure and then pulled posteriorly. In this way, the mucosa over the cord can be stripped. A laryngeal suction tube may be placed over the ventricular surface of the cord so that when the cord is pushed downwards, the mucosa is rolled on the undersurface medially. In this way the mucosa on the undersurface can be stripped adequately under direct vision (Fig. 2.3). Once carcinoma in-situ is confirmed by pathological examination of the specimen, the patient should be followed up closely with endoscopic examination, and further stripping performed for any suspicious recurrent lesion.

Carbon dioxide laser resection

Carbon dioxide (CO_2) laser is the most frequently used laser for laryngeal surgery. It has a wavelength of 10.6 μm and its energy is absorbed by water. As soft tissue of the body has a high water content, the energy delivered with the CO_2 laser is concentrated to where it is delivered, rather than being dissipated to the surrounding tissue.

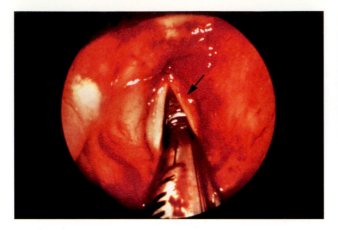

Figure 2.3 Endoscopic view of the vocal cord after stripping of the overlying mucosa and the early carcinoma (arrow).

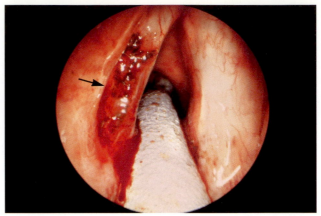

Figure 2.4 Endoscopic view of the vocal cord after CO_2 laser excision of an early carcinoma of the larynx (arrow).

This rapid fall in energy leads to predictable tissue incision, with minimal tissue oedema. The CO_2 laser has limited haemostatic ability when it is applied for incision, but when it is used in a defocus form, it can coagulate vessels of up to 1 mm in diameter. These characteristics make the CO_2 laser a precise cutting instrument in a relatively bloodless field. It is ideal for performing excision of small lesions over a delicate structure such as the vocal cord.

As CO_2 laser cannot be transmitted through flexible endoscopes, a rigid delivery system with mirrors has to be used. This can be coupled with the operating microscope and also with the micromanipulator; thus, CO_2 laser may be delivered on the vocal cord through the operating microscope at a spot size of 0.3 mm. For the excision of early carcinoma of the vocal cords, an energy of 2–3 W with the pulse mode set at a 0.1-second interval should be used.

Laser excision of early laryngeal carcinoma is carried out under general anaesthesia using endotracheal intubation. In view of the risk of the laser beam damaging the endotracheal tube, a metallic type of tube or the routinely used endotracheal tube should be wrapped with a shiny strapping to reflect away the light energy. Otherwise, ventilation of the patient may be maintained with the tubeless high-frequency jet ventilation technique. The larynx may be exposed as in microlaryngoscopy and the whole laryngeal inlet thoroughly examined under magnification to determine the lesion to be treated. Toluidine blue may be administered to stain the dysplastic mucosa so that the extent of the resection may be determined precisely. With toluidine blue, dysplastic mucosa is stained dark blue, in contrast to normal mucosa [9]. Once the lesion to be excised has been decided upon, the laser spot is guided around the lesion until the entire circular incision is completed. The mucosa over the vocal cord, with the lesion in the centre, may be lifted with a microforceps. This piece of mucosa may then be dissected away from the vocalis muscle, either by using microscissors or directly with the CO_2 laser (Fig. 2.4). The specimen should be removed in one piece and sent for pathological examination.

Laser cordectomy may also be performed endoscopically for T1 cancer of the vocal cord. Under these circumstances, the incision with the CO_2 laser penetrates to the vocalis muscle such that, by using a lateral incision, the segment of the cord bearing the lesion may be removed completely. Such an incision should spare both the anterior commissure and the arytenoid cartilage.

Treatment of early cancer of the glottis with CO_2 laser provides results that are comparable with those obtained after radiotherapy; moreover, the laser operation may be completed in one session. When laser treatment is correctly performed, the quality of voice postoperatively is not inferior to that in patients treated with radiotherapy. The disadvantages of CO_2 laser endoscopic surgery are two-fold:

- There is relatively poor tissue healing after excision of the lesion when compared with surgical excision, as the surgery is conducted with thermal energy.
- The capital cost of acquiring the laser machine, together with its maintenance, may not be cost-effective if it is not used frequently.

However, when the CO_2 laser technique is perfected, its use permits the precise excision of localized lesion over the vocal cords under magnification, and in a bloodless field.

Conservative surgery

The aim of conservative surgery is to remove the laryngeal cancer adequately, while at the same time preserving laryngeal function (Box 2.3). Conservative surgery may be performed as an oncological procedure because there are barriers in the larynx that prevent the spread of tumour from one side to the other, and from the upper regions of the larynx to the lower. Thus, resection is possible in either the vertical or the horizontal plane, as determined by the location of the tumour (Fig. 2.5). The exact extent of resection may only be decided at the time of surgery, using frozen section control. As the intra-operative extent of resection may well exceed the original planned limit, consent must be obtained for total laryngectomy in all patients undergoing conservative resection.

Patient selection for conservative surgery is important for a favourable outcome. All patients will have a tracheostomy on completion of surgery. With subsequent training and adaptation, decannulation is possible in over 90% of patients if the selection has been appropriate.

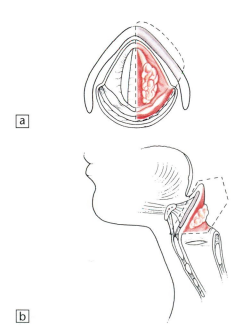

Figure 2.5 Schematic drawing of the extent of resection (broken line) for (a) vertical hemilaryngectomy and (b) horizontal hemilaryngectomy.

Elderly patients with neurological disease may find it difficult to adapt to the poor voice and the aspiration on swallowing. Patients with chronic pulmonary problems are also not suitable, as their pulmonary reserve may be unable to tolerate the significant aspiration, especially during the early postoperative period. It has been shown that when the forced expiratory volume in 1 second to forced vital capacity ($FEV_1 : FVC$) ratio is less than 50% of the predicted value then there is an increased morbidity following aspiration [10].

Vertical hemilaryngectomy

This is most frequently used for glottic carcinoma which affects one vocal cord. The extent of the hemilaryngectomy depends on the extent of the tumour.

Cordectomy (laryngofissure)

This is suitable for small carcinoma confined to the superficial part of the vocal cord, such as T1 and T2 carcinoma, the posterior extent of which has not reached the vocal process of the arytenoid cartilage. This is also applicable in the occasional post-radiotherapy failure patients in whom recurrent or persistent disease is minor and localized. In laryngofissure, the resection is confined to the mucosa and submucosal soft tissue. Laryngeal cartilage is not removed with the tumour.

Most of these carcinomas are currently managed with endoscopic resection, either with the application of CO_2 laser or with scissors and microblades. When these facilities are unavailable, or when the anatomical structure of the patient prevents full exposure of the laryngeal inlet for the endoscopic procedure, then an open approach is applicable. This procedure is not suitable when the laryngeal carcinoma has subglottic extension or involves the ventricles.

The surgical procedure for cordectomy begins with a tracheostomy. This allows ventilation of the patient without having to place an endotracheal tube in the larynx that might interfere with tumour identification and resection. The thyroid cartilage is divided precisely along the midline so that the perichondrium on the inner aspect of the thyroid cartilage is not disturbed. This procedure may be achieved satisfactorily with an oscillating saw, using a small blade. After retraction of the thyroid cartilage, the cricothyroid membrane and the thyrohyoid membrane are also incised so that the upper and lower extent of the tumour may be identified. The mucosal lining above and below the cord is excised with the tumour-bearing vocal cord. The posterior limit of division of the cord is in front of the vocal process of the arytenoid cartilage (Fig. 2.6).

The thyroid cartilage is then returned so that there is no need for glottic reconstruction. The damaged area heals by re-epithelialization, and thus a functional 'pseudo vocal cord' is formed. In order to produce a better postoperative voice, a strip of the central portion of the thyroid cartilage may be removed so that the remaining opposite cord can be sutured closer to the returned thyroid cartilage; this results in better phonation.

Possible complications of this approach include early atelectasis, perichondritis and late laryngeal web formation or stenosis. Some patients may also develop sequestrum of the cartilage, though fortunately the incidence of this complication is low among non-irradiated patients [11]. Cordectomy has been used to control local tumour successfully in 60% to 98% of patients, depending on the number of those who have undergone previous radiotherapy [11–13].

Frontolateral partial laryngectomy

The concept of laryngofissure may be extended for the treatment of the slightly larger glottic tumours that cross the anterior commissure to the other vocal cord yet remain localized at the glottic level (Fig. 2.7).

A segment of the thyroid cartilage is removed, together with a varying length of the anterior portion of both vocal cords in order to effect tumour clearance (Figs 2.8, 2.9). When less than one-third of the vocal cord is removed, part of the laryngeal mucosa may be mobilized

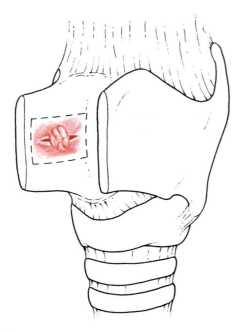

Figure 2.6 Schematic drawing of the extent of cordectomy (broken line), with splitting of the thyroid cartilage in the midline.

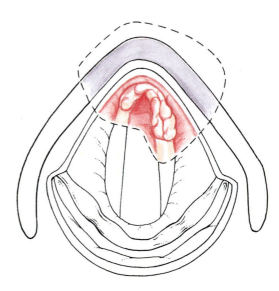

Figure 2.7 Schematic drawing of the extent of frontolateral partial laryngectomy (broken line).

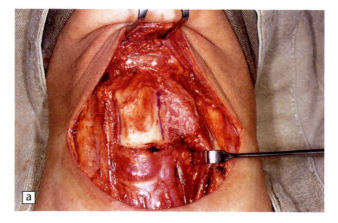

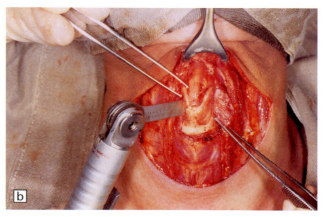

Figure 2.8 (a) Intraoperative photograph showing the incision on the thyroid cartilage to enter the larynx for frontolateral partial laryngectomy. (b) Showing saw cut on thyroid cartilage to enter the larynx during frontolateral partial laryngectomy.

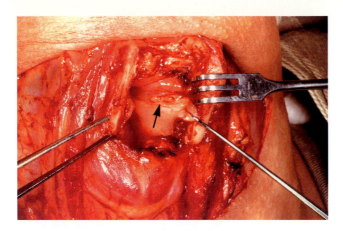

Figure 2.9 During frontolateral laryngectomy, the tumour (arrow) is seen after entering the larynx.

for reconstruction of the vocal cord. When more tissue is included in the resection, some form of reconstruction such as a skin graft or bipedicled strap muscle flap should be used. Good results have been reported using a temporary partition stent which is inserted between the divided thyroid cartilage to allow mucosal healing on either side [14]. The 3-year cure rate reported following frontolateral partial laryngectomy in suitable patients was about 70% [14,15].

Vertical hemilaryngectomy

Anatomically, vertical hemilaryngectomy removes one vocal cord from the anterior commissure to include the arytenoid cartilage in the coronal plane and the vocal cord with its overlying mucosa, the ipsilateral false cord, ventricle, the paraglottic space, the aryepiglottic fold and the overlying thyroid cartilage in the sagittal plane. Vertical hemilaryngectomy is applicable for T2 and limited T3 carcinoma of the vocal cord. As long as the supraglottic extension is up to the false cords and the subglottic extension is less than 5 mm, then vertical hemilaryngectomy is feasible. Fixation of the vocal cord is not a contraindication as long as the limited mobility is not due to extensive subglottic infiltration or fixation of the cricoarytenoid joint.

As the surgical procedure compromises the laryngeal airway, its function of vocalization and protection of the airway, reconstructive procedures are necessary to ensure an adequate laryngeal passage, a functional glottic voice, and also protection of the airway during deglutition.

Thorough preoperative endoscopic examination is essential to assess the operability and also to determine where to enter the larynx. A tracheostomy is performed at the start of the operation so that the endotracheal tube is removed to allow an unobstructed view of the endolarynx. The laryngeal skeleton is exposed by retracing the strap muscles, preserving their neurovascular bundle.

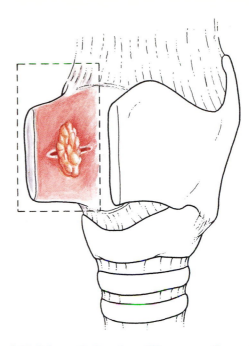

Figure 2.10 Schematic drawing of the extent of resection of vertical hemilaryngectomy (broken line) after the larynx is entered from the front.

The outer pericondrium of the thyroid cartilage is first elevated, after which the larynx is entered through an incision on the cartilage either in the midline or to one side, contralateral to the carcinoma. The cricothyroid membrane is incised and extended horizontally along the superior border of the cricoid cartilage to allow adequate examination of the subglottic region. Similarly, the thyrohyoid membrane is incised and extended laterally along the superior border of the thyroid cartilage to release the epiglottis superiorly. After these incisions have been made, the involved half of the larynx may be rotated laterally to expose the cancer completely. With the cancer under direct vision, a second vertical incision is placed on the thyroid cartilage behind the lesion so that the entire tumour is removed with a good margin (Fig. 2.10). This incision should leave about 1 cm of the posterior border of the thyroid cartilage on the side of the tumour. The attachment of the inferior constrictor to this part of the thyroid cartilage should be left intact to provide tissue for reconstruction.

When the anterior commissure has been removed, the anterior remnant of the cord may be sutured to the preserved thyroid outer perichondrium. The glottis is reconstructed by rotating a pedicled strap muscle into the larynx, while the arytenoid cartilage on the side of the cancer may be reconstructed with a segment of the preserved posterior rim of the thyroid cartilage.

Complications related to the operation are infrequent, and decannulation is rarely a problem. Although postoperatively the resultant voice is often hoarse and not too strong, voice rehabilitation is better than after total laryngectomy. In selected patients, vertical hemilaryngectomy may effect a cure rate of 80% for T2 carcinoma, and 60% for T3 [16–18].

Horizontal laryngectomy

Supraglottic horizontal laryngectomy

Many supraglottic carcinomas are exophytic, well-circumscribed, and involve the region above the anterior commissure. When these tumours do not involve the vocal cord, they may be removed with the supraglottic horizontal laryngectomy. Under these circumstances, a narrow margin of uninvolved mucosa is adequate for control of the tumour. Surgery involves removal of the whole epiglottis, the aryepiglottic fold, the pre-epiglottic space, the false cords and the upper part of the thyroid cartilage. Essentially, all the laryngeal structures above the vocal cords are removed. However, the hyoid bone is not removed, except in extensive disease. This procedure is suitable for T1 or T2 carcinoma of the supraglottic region (Fig. 2.11).

Detailed endoscopic examination of the larynx before surgery is again essential to assess the extent of tumour, and also to determine the location of the point of entry to the larynx. A tracheostomy is performed first, after which the upper portion of the thyroid cartilage is exposed. The perichondrium over the thyroid cartilage is lifted and preserved. The incision on the thyroid cartilage should be just above the level of the anterior commissure, and this marks the lower limit of the resection. The neurovascular pedicle of the superior laryngeal vessels should be preserved to maintain the sensation of the mucosa that is preserved. The lumen of the oropharynx is entered by incision through the vallecula, if this is not involved by tumour (Fig. 2.12). The epiglottis is then grasped and the aryepiglottic fold divided bilaterally. The epiglottis with the cancer is then turned anteroinferiorly and the supraglottic laryngectomy can be completed. After ensuring that the margin of resection is clear, the laryngeal remnant is sutured to the base of the tongue.

To facilitate recovery and prevention of aspiration, the larynx may be suspended with interrupted sutures to the inferior border of the mandible. A cricomyotomy may be carried out to reduce the hypopharyngeal resistance to swallowing, and this lessens the chance of aspiration. The vallecula and the base of the tongue, when involved by tumour, may also be removed with this supraglottic laryngectomy.

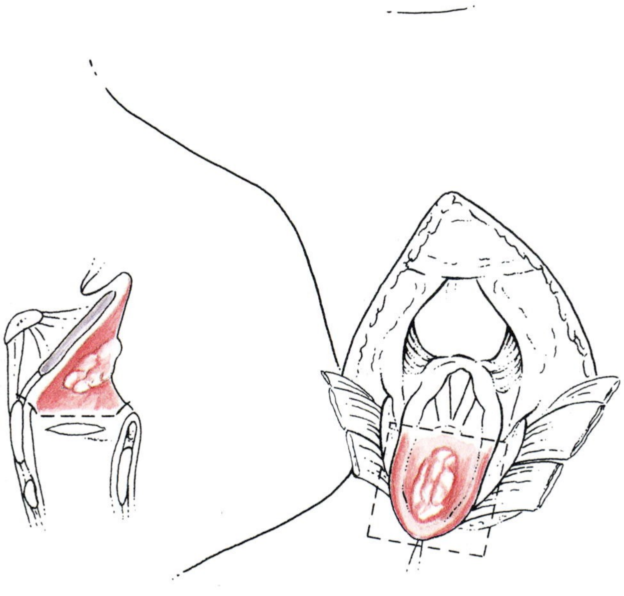

Figure 2.11 Schematic drawing of the extent of resection of horizontal hemilaryngectomy (broken line) after the larynx is entered from the vallecula.

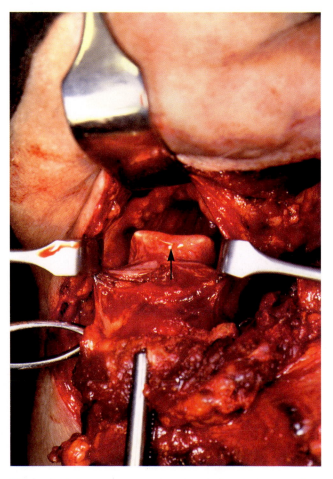

Figure 2.12 Intraoperative photograph showing entry of the oropharynx through the vallecula. The tip of the epiglottis is just visible (arrow).

Nearly all patients suffer from some degree of aspiration soon after the operation, although most are able to swallow effectively after 1–2 months. The tumour control rate with the supraglottic horizontal laryngectomy is around 75%, which is comparable with that seen after radiotherapy [19,20].

Summary

The aim of treatment for early carcinoma of the larynx is eradication of tumour, while simultaneously preserving laryngeal function. For most early cancers, this may be achieved with radiotherapy alone, though for patients who are unsuitable for radiotherapy surgical extirpation provides similar results. The choice of the surgical options depends on the size and location of the tumour, and also whether the tumour can be exposed adequately with the endoscope. The least traumatic approach to provide eradication of the tumour should be employed, as the preservation of laryngeal function is inversely proportional to the amount of tissue removed.

References

1. Mendenhall WM, Parsons JT, Stringer SP *et al*. Carcinoma of the supraglottic larynx: a basis for comparing the results of radiotherapy and surgery. *Head Neck* 1990; 12: 204–209.

2. Harwood AR, Beale FA, Cummins BJ *et al*. Supraglottic laryngeal carcinoma: an analysis of dose-time-volume factors in 410 patients. *Int J Radiat Oncol Biol Phys* 1983; 9: 311–319.

3. Spaulding CA, Krochak RJ, Hahn SS, Constable WC. Radiotherapeutic management of cancer of the supraglottis. *Cancer* 1986; 57: 1292–1298.

4. Mendenhall WM, Million RR. Elective neck irradiation for squamous cell carcinoma of the head and neck: analysis of time-dose factors and causes of failure. *Int J Radiat Oncol Biol Phys* 1986; 12: 741–746.

5. Wang CC. Treatment of glottic carcinoma by megavoltage radiation therapy and results. *Am J Roentgenol* 1974; 120: 157–163.

6. Kelly MD, Hahn SS, Spaulding CA *et al*. Definitive radiotherapy in the management of stage I and II carcinoma of the glottis. *Ann Otol Rhinol Laryngol* 1989; 98: 235–239.

7. Small W, Jr, Mittal BB, Brand WN *et al*. Results of radiation therapy in early glottic carcinoma: multivariate analysis of prognostic and radiation therapy variables. *Radiology* 1992; 183: 789–794.

8. Guedea F, Parsons JT, Mendenhall WM *et al*. Primary subglottic cancer: results of radical radiation therapy. *Int J Radiat Oncol Biol Phys* 1992; 21: 1607–1611.

9. Strong M, Vaughan CW, Incze J. Toluidine blue in diagnosis of cancer of the larynx. *Arch Otolaryngol* 1970; 91: 515–519.

10. Beckhardt RN, Murray JG, Ford CN *et al*. Factors influencing functional outcome in supraglottic laryngectomy. *Head Neck* 1994; 16: 232–239.

11. Neel HB, Devine KD, Desanto LW. Laryngofissure and cordectomy for early cordal carcinoma: outcome in 182 patients. *Otolaryngol Head Neck Surg* 1980; 88: 79–84.

12. Daly JF, Kwok FN. Laryngofissure and cordectomy. *Laryngoscope* 1975; 85: 1290–1297.

13. Sessions DG, Manes GM, McSwain B. Laryngofissure in the treatment of carcinoma of the vocal cord: a report of forty cases and a review of the literature. *Laryngoscope* 1965; 75: 490–502.

14. Som ML, Silver CE. The anterior commissure technique of partial laryngectomy. *Arch Otolaryngol* 1968; 87: 138–145.

15. Kirchner JA, Som ML. The anterior commissure technique of partial laryngectomy: clinical and laboratory observations. *Laryngoscope* 1975; 85: 1308–1317.

16. Ogura JH, Sessions DG, Spector GJ. Analysis of surgical therapy for epidermoid carcinoma of the laryngeal glottis. *Laryngoscope* 1975; 85: 1522–1530.

17. Leroux-Robert J. A statistical study of 620 laryngeal carcinomas of the glottic region personally operated upon more than five years ago. *Laryngoscope* 1975; 85: 1440–1452.

18. Som ML. Cordal cancer with extension to vocal process. *Laryngoscope* 1975; 85: 1298–1307.

19. Bocca E, Pignataro O, Oldini C *et al*. Supraglottic laryngectomy: 30 years of experience. *Ann Otol Rhinol Laryngol* 1983; 92: 14–18.

20. Ogura JH, Sessions DG, Spector GJ. Conservation surgery for epidermoid carcinoma of the supraglottic larynx. *Laryngoscope* 1975; 85: 1808–1815.

CHAPTER three

Management of advanced
laryngeal cancer

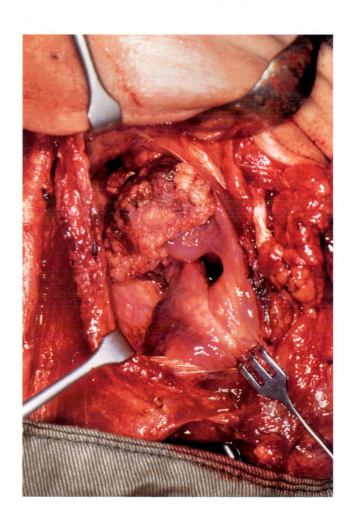

Introduction

When laryngeal carcinoma is so advanced that it cannot be adequately managed by partial laryngectomy, then a more extensive surgical resection is necessary. Surgical management options for advanced laryngeal carcinoma include supracricoid laryngectomy, near-total laryngectomy and total laryngectomy (Table 3.1).

Surgical treatment options

Supracricoid laryngectomy

Overview

When the main tumour is located in the supraglottic region and extends down to affect the vocal cords anteriorly, then horizontal supraglottic partial laryngectomy will not suffice and an extended resection is necessary for the eradication of tumour.

When the tumour does not affect the epiglottis, then resection of the whole thyroid cartilage, both false and true vocal cords, one arytenoid cartilage and the paraglottic space should be carried out for tumour extirpation. Reconstruction may be performed with cricohyoidoepiglottopexy, i.e. suturing the lower portion of the epiglottis to the cricoid cartilage anteriorly and also the remaining arytenoid cartilage on the posterior aspect [1] (Fig. 3.1).

When laryngeal carcinoma affects the epiglottis, then it can be removed completely with the pre-epiglottic space. The whole thyroid cartilage together with both false and true cords may also be resected to ensure a good margin of tumour clearance. One or both arytenoids can be preserved, depending on the location of the tumour.

The laryngeal apparatus is then reconstructed by suturing the hyoid to the cricoid cartilage, i.e. cricohyoidopexy [2] (Fig. 3.2).

Surgical techniques (see Box 3.1)

The operation is performed with transoral endotracheal intubation. The strap muscles are lifted from the laryngeal skeleton and the superior laryngeal vessels are divided. The piriform mucosa is lifted off the inner aspect of the thyroid cartilage and the cricoid is separated from the thyroid cartilage. Care is exercised to preserve the recurrent laryngeal nerve, at least on one side, together with the arytenoid cartilage. The pharynx is entered below the hyoid bone and the pharyngeal incision is made along the side of the thyroid cartilage with the tumour under direct vision (Fig. 3.3). After removing the tumour the cricoid cartilage, with at least one arytenoid, is sutured to the base of the tongue, or the epiglottis if it is not removed. Temporary tracheostomy is performed on completion of surgery. The morbidity associated with the operation is low, and nearly all patients can be decannulated [2]. Most patients are able to tolerate an oral diet one month after surgery.

Box 3.1 *Strategic manoeuvres during supracricoid laryngectomy*

- Strap muscle preserved
- Superior laryngeal vessels and nerves divided
- One recurrent laryngeal nerve and one arytenoid cartilage on same side preserved
- Preserve piriform fossa mucosa
- Temporary tracheostomy

Table 3.1 *Surgical options for treatment of advanced carcinoma of the larynx*

	Supracricoid laryngectomy	Near-total laryngectomy	Total laryngectomy
Location of tumour	One arytenoid and subglottic region free of tumour	One arytenoid not involved by tumour	Tumour within the laryngeal skeleton
Cricoid cartilage preserved	Yes	No	No
Other laryngeal cartilages preserved	One arytenoid with or without epiglottis	One arytenoid	No
Permanent tracheostomy	No	Yes	Yes
Postoperative speech	Laryngeal speech	Occlusion of tracheostomy to produce speech	Oesophageal or other types of alaryngeal speech

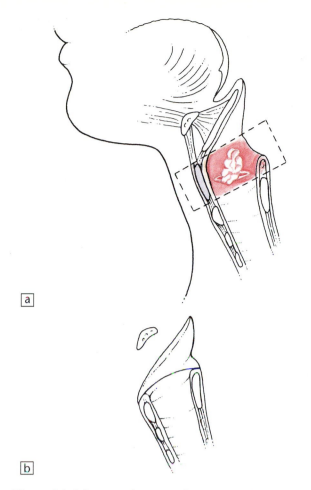

Figure 3.1 Schematic drawing of supracricoid laryngectomy with cricohyoidoepiglottopexy. (a) Extent of resection (broken line). (b) Reconstruction.

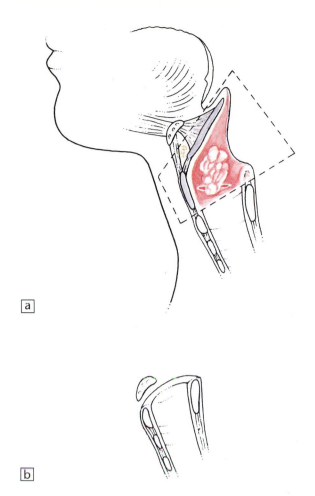

Figure 3.2 Schematic drawing of supracricoid laryngectomy with cricohyoidopexy. (a) Extent of resection (broken line). (b) Reconstruction.

Supracricoid laryngectomy is indicated for supraglottic carcinoma which involves the vocal cords, including the anterior commissure with impaired cord mobility. It is also applicable for T3 transglottic carcinomas which involve the anterior part of the vocal cords, thus affecting their mobility, as well as for some T4 cancers which have involved a localized area of the thyroid cartilage. This procedure is contraindicated when the tumour affects the cricoid cartilage, the hyoid bone or the base of the tongue. If there is subglottic extension of greater than 1 cm or when the arytenoids are fixed, then this operation should not be performed.

Near-total laryngectomy

Overview

When the carcinoma is localized to one side of the larynx, it is possible to perform an extended hemilaryngectomy to eradicate the tumour. The resection should include the cricoid cartilage, both vocal cords, the epiglottis and also the perilaryngeal tissue. This operation – first proposed by Pearson in 1980 – was termed 'near-total laryngectomy' [3]. After resection, the mucosa retained is not able to provide an adequate airway, thus a permanent tracheostomy is necessary. A mucosa-lined tracheo-pharyngeal shunt can be created to allow provision for vocalization. One arytenoid cartilage and the recurrent laryngeal nerve on the same side are preserved to form part of the dynamic phonetic shunt (Fig. 3.4). This procedure allows oncological resection of the tumour with the restoration of lung-powered speech while aspiration during swallowing is prevented [4]. The prerequisite for this operative procedure is that the posterior commissure and one arytenoid must be free from tumour.

Surgical technique (see Box 3.2)

A tracheostomy is performed at the start of the operation to avoid the need for an endotracheal tube in the laryngeal lumen. The larynx is mobilized as for total laryngectomy and the laryngeal cartilage on the contralateral side to the tumour is skeletonized. The pharynx is entered

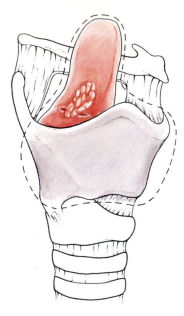

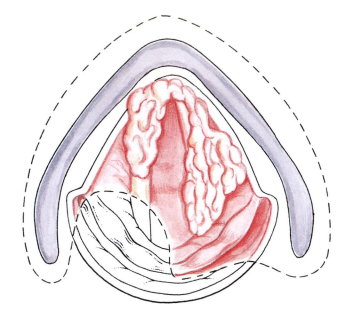

Figure 3.3 Schematic drawing of supracricoid laryngectomy showing the extent of resection (broken line) after entering the pharynx from below the hyoid bone.

Figure 3.4 Schematic drawing of near-total laryngectomy showing the extent of resection (broken line).

> **Box 3.2** *Strategic manoeuvres during near-total laryngectomy*
>
> - Tracheostomy carried out before resection
> - Entire tumour resected under direct vision
> - One arytenoid cartilage and recurrent nerve situated contralateral to the tumour is preserved
> - Mucosa over piriform fossa and the postcricoid region is preserved
> - Mucosal tube for vocalization is constructed over a 14 Fr tube

above the hyoid bone and the exact location of the tumour determined. The thyroid and cricoid cartilages are included in the resection while the arytenoid and its accompanying recurrent laryngeal nerve are preserved. Mucosa over the inner aspect of the cricoid cartilage is lifted, and together with some piriform sinus mucosa, is used to construct a mucosal tube. This shunt, of 14 Fr diameter, extends from the trachea to the pharynx with the remaining arytenoid guarding its pharyngeal entrance (Fig. 3.5). Initially, the patient is fed via a nasogastric tube, and when oral feeding starts phonation is possible with occlusion of the terminal tracheostomy.

The results of control of tumour with this operation are comparable with those of total laryngectomy. In a report of 225 patients, the local recurrence rate was 4% with at least 2-year follow-up. More than 85% of patients were able to use the fistula for vocalization, and postoperative

radiotherapy did not affect the function of the speaking shunt [5]. In suitable patients, near-total laryngectomy is considered an appropriate alternative to total laryngectomy without compromising the tumour clearance.

Total laryngectomy

Overview

The operation of total laryngectomy removes all the structures of the larynx, including the pre-epiglottic and paraglottic spaces. Breathing and swallowing involve different parts of the aerodigestive tract as the pharynx is completely separated from the trachea and thus ventilation is possible through a permanent tracheostomy. Although the first total laryngectomy was performed by Billroth in 1873 [6], in the first half of the 20th century, radiotherapy was frequently employed for the treatment of cancer of the larynx. Surgical and anaesthetic techniques have improved significantly in recent years, while the limitations of radiotherapy are universally being recognized. Surgical treatment for cancer of the larynx, including total laryngectomy, continues to play a substantial role.

With the introduction of the various types of conservative laryngectomy, the frequency of total laryngectomy for treatment of carcinoma of the larynx has declined. This is particularly attributed to the introduction of near-total laryngectomy with retention of vocalization ability without jeopardizing cure. Despite these considerations, total laryngectomy for laryngeal cancer remains as the standard against which other operations and treatment modalities are judged with regard to cure rates.

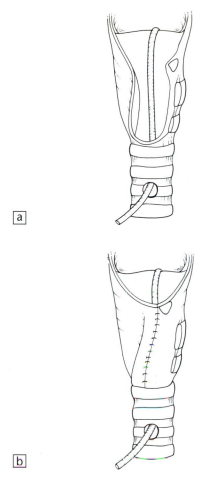

Figure 3.5 Schematic drawing of reconstruction of the mucosal tube following near-total laryngectomy. (a) Posterior tracheal wall is exposed, continuity with pharynx is maintained through the posterior commissure, guarded by one arytenoid cartilage. (b) Tracheal mucosal tube constructed by suturing over a 14 Fr tube with the inner end placed within the pharynx and other end brought out through the tracheostomy. The arytenoid cartilage guards the upper end of the mucosal tube.

The indications for total laryngectomy are:

- Related to the primary tumour:
  a. Advanced carcinoma of the larynx with destruction of cartilage with or without extralaryngeal spread.
  b. Tumour involvement of the posterior commissure, the arytenoids or extensive subglottic extension that precludes other forms of conservative laryngectomy.
  c. Hypopharyngeal carcinoma involving the larynx or, upon removal of the tumour, the motor function of the larynx is likely to be affected.
  d. Advanced (non-squamous) malignancy of the larynx which does not respond to radiotherapy, e.g. sarcoma, minor salivary gland tumour and adenocarcinoma.

- Related to the patient:
  a. Elderly and debilitated patients whose general condition and pulmonary reserve precludes a hazardous postoperative course following conservative laryngectomy.
  b. Patients living in remote areas where close follow-up to monitor recurrence after conservative laryngectomy is not possible.
  c. Completion total laryngectomy when conservative surgery is not successful, e.g. when there is significant aspiration following initial surgery.
- As salvage therapy:
  a. Post-radiotherapy recurrence when the tumour is T2 or higher stage.
  b. Local recurrence after conservative laryngectomy.

Surgical technique (see Box 3.3)

The operation is performed under general anaesthesia. Initially, ventilation of the patient is maintained via endotracheal intubation. Insertion of the endotracheal tube may be difficult when there is gross tumour situated at the laryngeal inlet, but this problem may be overcome with the use of a flexible endoscope. An appropriate-sized endotracheal tube is railroaded onto a flexible bronchoscope as a sheath. An ordinary 5.9 mm-tip bronchoscope can comfortably be inserted into a number 7.5 mm diameter cuffed endotracheal tube. When the use of a smaller diameter endotracheal tube is necessary, a paediatric bronchoscope must be used. The bronchoscope is inserted through the nasal passage, the nasopharynx and the oropharynx. Once the tumour is seen at the laryngeal inlet, the tip of the bronchoscope can be manipulated to bypass the tumour for insertion into the trachea, beyond the lower limit of the tumour. The endotracheal tube may then be advanced into the trachea with the bronchoscope as the stylet [7,8]. Correct positioning of the tip of the endotracheal tube is checked with the bronchoscope.

> **Box 3.3** *Strategic manoeuvres during total laryngectomy*
>
> - Transverse neck incision with separate 'X-shaped' incision for terminal tracheostome
> - Remove the lobe of the thyroid gland on the side where the tumour involves the glottic or subglottic region
> - Enter the pharynx from the region furthest from the tumour
> - Pharyngeal mucosa must be 3 cm wide before primary closure is carried out
> - Pharyngeal closure in 'T' fashion with a reinforcing stitch at the 'T' junction

A transverse incision along the skin crease is adequate for exposure of the whole larynx. The neck incision is usually placed at the midpoint between the suprasternal notch and the upper border of the hyoid bone. The incision can be extended laterally when a larger flap needs to be elevated. With this transverse incision, the terminal tracheostomy wound can be placed at a separate, lower site (Fig. 3.6). When radical neck dissection has to be carried out at the same time, this transverse incision is carried laterally as the upper wound of the MacFee incision. Another parallel incision is placed over and along the clavicle as the lower surgical wound.

The larynx is mobilized after dividing the strap muscles and insertion of the inferior constrictor to the thyroid cartilage. The neurovascular supply of the larynx, and the superior laryngeal nerves and vessels are divided before they enter the thyrohyoid membrane (Fig. 3.7). After dividing the sternohyoid and sternothyroid muscles, the thyroid gland is exposed. The isthmus of the thyroid gland is divided and retracted laterally to expose the trachea down to the sternal notch. With blunt dissection, the trachea is separated from the oesophagus posteriorly. The cuff of the endotracheal tube should be deflated to avoid overdistension and thinning of the posterior tracheal wall, thus lowering the risk of its being damaged. The recurrent laryngeal nerve is identified in the tracheo-oesophageal groove and divided.

One lobe of the thyroid gland should be removed with the larynx when the primary laryngeal carcinoma is stage T4, or when the tumour exhibits subglottic involvement. Whole organ section studies of the resected laryngeal specimens have shown that for patients with these features, there is a high incidence of involvement of the thyroid gland by laryngeal carcinoma [9]. Hemithyroidectomy has low early postoperative and long-term morbidity. It is recommended for tumour clearance for T4 carcinoma and for those tumours that involve the subglottic region. Total thyroidectomy should be carried out when the tumour has invaded the thyroid gland

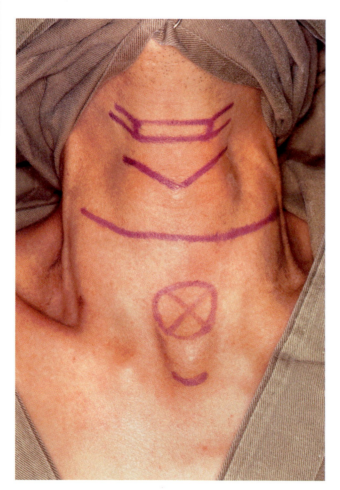

Figure 3.6 Transverse incision for total laryngectomy. The terminal tracheostomy site is placed at a separate location.

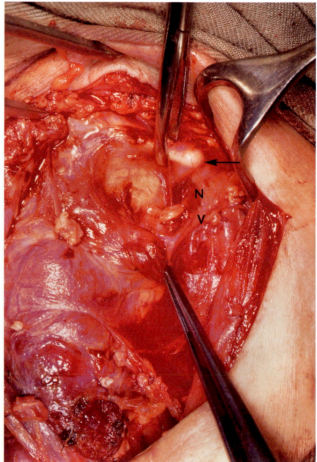

Figure 3.7 The superior laryngeal nerve (N) and vessel (V) are identified and divided below the greater cornu of the hyoid bone (arrow).

macroscopically, or when both subglottic regions are involved. Total thyroidectomy should also be performed when laryngeal carcinoma has eroded the thyroid cartilage across the midline. The parathyroid gland should be preserved if possible, but attempts to do this should not jeopardize tumour clearance.

The terminal tracheostomy is created by dividing the trachea and suturing the lower end to a separate skin opening. The trachea is divided by an oblique incision to increase the diameter of the tracheostomy and to prevent later stenosis. As a circular mucocutaneous apposition tends to contract concentrically and thus lead to stenosis, modifications of the construction of the terminal tracheostomy have been suggested. The skin incision for the terminal tracheostomy is designed to be X-shaped rather than the conventional circular incision, thus creating four triangular flaps (Fig. 3.8). Four vertical slits are also made on the anterior, lateral and posterior walls of the trachea. These incisions should divide at least two tracheal rings, after which the four skin flaps can be inset into these slits. This will result in a serrated tracheocutaneous suture line (Fig. 3.9), and any contraction of the wound will tend to open up the tracheostomy rather than lead to stenosis [10]. The incidence of tracheostomy stenosis following total laryngectomy is greatly reduced with this technique [11].

Once the trachea is divided, ventilation of the patient can only be carried out through a tracheostomy tube inserted into the lower end of the divided trachea. Suturing of the trachea to the surrounding skin is sometimes hampered by the bulky tracheostomy tube, and this is particularly so when a serrated mucocutaneous suturing line is being created. A ventilation jet connected to a metal tube may be used to maintain ventilation of the patient during construction of the tracheostomy [12]. On completion of the terminal tracheostomy, ventilation via the tracheostomy tube is resumed.

After construction of the terminal tracheostomy, the pharynx mucosa must be incised to expose the larynx. There are different ways of entering the pharynx. One approach is to open the pharynx from above the hyoid bone; under these circumstances the hyoid bone is stabilized with a pair of forceps and the base of the tongue muscle is divided above it until the vallecular mucosa is incised. This approach of entering the pharynx in the midline avoids cutting into those tumours that are situated at a lower level. It also allows visualization of the postcricoid area before resection is carried out in the region. An alternative approach is to enter the pharynx from the side by dividing the inferior constrictor muscle and then the pharyngeal mucosa behind the thyroid cartilage (Fig. 3.10). This method is useful when the primary laryngeal carcinoma involves the supraglottic region or affects the epiglottis.

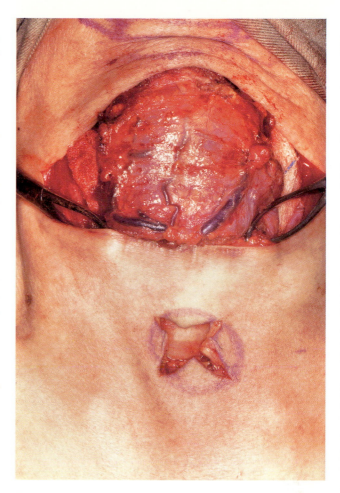

Figure 3.8 The skin incision for the terminal tracheostomy is X-shaped, and this results in four skin flaps to be inset into the vertical slits of the trachea.

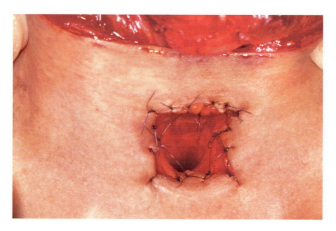

Figure 3.9 The completed terminal tracheostomy with the serrated tracheocutaneous suture line.

Thus, the route of entry to the pharynx for removing the larynx depends on the location of the primary tumour [13]. When the main bulk is in the lower segment of the larynx, or is located in the posterior aspect and affects the arytenoids, then the superior entry should be used. If the tumour is located in the upper portion, such as the supraglottic region, or erodes the epiglottis, then the lateral entry on the side opposite to the main tumour should be employed. By selecting the appropriate approach for the individual patient, adequate tumour removal may be achieved with direct visualization of the tumour.

After the tumour has been removed with the larynx, the remnant pharyngeal mucosa may be closed primarily when there is adequate mucosal tissue available. When a supraglottic tumour extends into the surrounding pharyngeal wall, then some pharyngeal mucosa must be removed for tumour clearance. It has been shown that when the mean width of the remaining pharyngeal wall is more than 3.2 cm when relaxed and 4.8 cm when stretched, then the neopharynx can be reconstructed without risk of future stenosis [14]. When more pharyngeal mucosa is removed, a separate flap is required to augment the pharyngeal lumen (Fig. 3.11).

As the shape of the cut edge of the pharynx after total laryngectomy is a triangle, the most appropriate way of suturing the neopharynx is in a T-shaped fashion. The greatest tension is usually at the junction of the two suture lines. An extra interrupted three-point stitch should be added to reduce tissue tension and facilitate healing. A nasogastric tube is inserted for feeding during the early postoperative period. In patients where a tracheo-oesophageal puncture is created for voice prosthesis insertion, a feeding tube may be inserted through this tract, thus avoiding the discomfort associated with tube insertion via the nostril.

Results

For surgical treatment alone in the form of total laryngectomy, when carried out for T3N0 supraglottic laryngeal carcinoma, the cure rate was reported as 53%; when performed for T4N0 carcinoma the rate was 52% [15]. When surgery is employed for T3N0 glottic carcinoma, the 5-year actuarial survival rate was 80% [16]. For

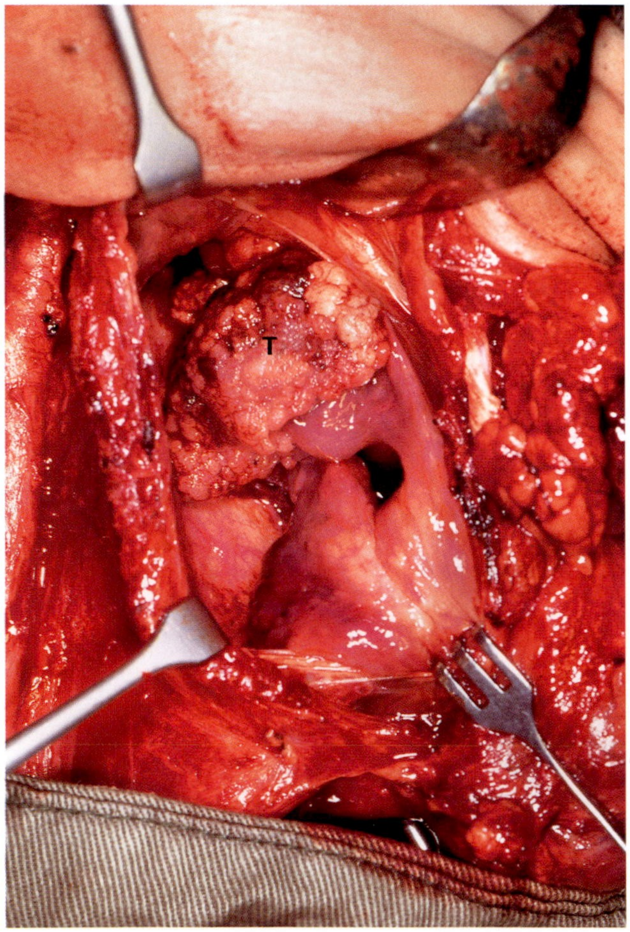

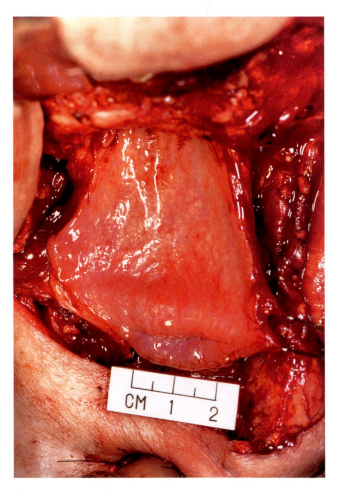

Figure 3.10 The pharynx is entered from the behind the thyroid cartilage to avoid cutting into a tumour located at the supraglottic region (T).

Figure 3.11 The pharyngeal remnant after total laryngectomy must be at least 3.2 cm wide when stretched before a primary closure can be carried out without functional disturbance.

patients who developed tumour recurrence after radical radiotherapy, total laryngectomy was shown to achieve a salvage rate of 65% [17].

The concept of laryngeal preservation

In the past, the recognized standard treatment for localized advanced laryngeal cancer has been surgery followed by radiotherapy. The most frequently employed surgical treatment in this context is total laryngectomy. Although such surgery is successful in eradicating cancer, many patients are unable to acquire adequate speech ability postoperatively. Induction chemotherapy has not been found to improve survival rates in cancer of the larynx [18], but it may play an important role in the preservation of laryngeal function in these patients.

A phase II study was carried out in 64 patients suffering from resectable advanced head and neck cancer that affected the larynx. Each patient was given induction chemotherapy which included cisplatin and 5-fluorouracil (with or without bleomycin), followed by definitive radiotherapy to the primary tumour. Surgical resection was only carried out for those patients who did not respond to the chemotherapy, or as a salvage procedure. Those patients with laryngeal cancer had a 2-year survival rate of 71%, and 44% of the group had preservation of laryngeal function [19].

Clearer evidence was provided in a prospective randomized study of 332 patients with untreated advanced stage laryngeal cancer. These patients were assigned randomly to either three cycles of induction chemotherapy using cisplatin and 5-fluorouracil followed by radiotherapy, or to radical surgery (mostly total laryngectomy with or without radical neck dissection) followed by radiotherapy. In those patients who did not respond to chemotherapy or in whom tumour recurred after completion of chemotherapy and radiotherapy, surgery was performed as a salvage. The median follow-up of all patients was 33 months, and the 2-year survival rate was the same in both groups, 68%. The larynx was preserved in 64% of the patients receiving chemotherapy [20]. When this concept is applied to patients with advanced carcinoma of the larynx, close cooperation between the patient, the physician, and among the different disciplines of the medical profession is necessary before a favourable outcome is to be expected.

Summary

When the laryngeal tumour is extensive and limited resection is insufficient, then more radical surgery is mandatory for tumour eradication. The factors that affect the choice of operation are related to the extent of the primary tumour, the condition of the patient, and the timing of the operation, i.e. whether it is carried out as a salvage procedure or as primary treatment.

When the cricoid cartilage with one arytenoid and either the hyoid bone alone or together with the epiglottis can be preserved, then supracricoid laryngectomy should be performed. Thus, separation of the airway from the alimentary passage is not necessary and a terminal tracheostomy can be avoided. When only one arytenoid and the cricoid cartilage can be safely preserved, then near-total laryngectomy is the operation of choice. For all other advanced stage carcinoma of the larynx, total laryngectomy should be carried out. The fundamental goal is to remove the malignant growth completely, while preservation of function is considered secondary. Salient points of the surgical techniques involved are clearly presented in the text.

In recent years, the administration of induction chemotherapy with radiotherapy for advanced laryngeal cancer and surgical salvage as reserve has been shown to be possible in the conservation of laryngeal function in two-thirds of patients, without jeopardizing survival. However, close monitoring of these patients is mandatory if this treatment strategy is to be successful.

References

1. Piquet JJ, Chevalier D. Subtotal laryngectomy with crico-hyoido-epiglottopexy for the treatment of extended glottic carcinomas. *Am J Surg* 1991; 16: 357–361.

2. Laccourreye H, Laccourreye O, Weinstein G *et al*. Supracricoid laryngectomy with cricohyoidopexy: a partial laryngeal procedure for selected supraglottic and transglottic carcinomas. *Laryngoscope* 1990; 100: 735–741.

3. Pearson BW, Woods RD, Hartman DE. Extended hemilaryngectomy for T3 glottic carcinoma with preservation of speech and swallowing. *Laryngoscope* 1980; 90: 1950–1961.

4. Robbins K T, Michaels L. Feasibility of subtotal laryngectomy based on whole-organ examinations. *Arch Otolaryngol* 1985; 111: 356–360.

5. Pearson BW, De Santo LW, Olsen KD *et al*. Results of near-total laryngectomy. Ann Otol Rhinol Laryngol 1998.

6. Stell PM. The first laryngectomy for carcinoma. *Arch Otolaryngol* 1973; 98: 293.

7. Wei WI, Lau WF, Lam KH, Hui Y. The role of the fibreoptic bronchoscope in otorhinolaryngological practice. *J Laryngol Otol* 1987; 101: 1263–1270.

8. Wei WI, Siu KF, Lau WF, Lam KH. Emergency endotracheal intubation under fiberoptic endoscopic guidance for malignant laryngeal obstruction. *Otolaryngol Head Neck Surg* 1988; 98: 10–13.

9. Yuen APW, Wei WI, Lam KH, Ho CM. Thyroidectomy during laryngectomy for advanced laryngeal carcinoma – whole organ section study with long-term functional evaluation. *Clin Otolaryngol* 1995; 20: 145–149.

10. Lam KH, Wei WI, Wong J, Ong GB. Tracheostome construction during laryngectomy – a method to prevent stenosis. *Laryngoscope* 1983; 93: 212–215.

11. Ho CM, Wei WI, Lau WF, Lam KH. Tracheostomal stenosis after immediate tracheoesophageal puncture. *Arch Otolaryngol Head Neck Surg* 1991; 117: 662–665.

12. Chan ASH, Wei WI, Lau WF, Lam KH. Modified jet ventilation during total laryngectomy: a prospective study using pulse oximetry and a pressure regulator. *Anaesth Intens Care* 1990; 18: 504–508.

13. Wei WI, Lau WF, Lam KH. Entering the pharynx in total laryngectomy. *J Laryngol Otol* 1987; 101: 589–591.

14. Hui Y, Wei WI, Yuen PW *et al*. Primary closure of pharyngeal remnant after total laryngectomy and partial pharyngectomy: how much residual mucosa is sufficient. *Laryngoscope* 1996; 106: 490–494.

15. Alajmo E, Fini-Storchi O, Polli G. Five-year results of 1000 patients operated on for cancer of the larynx. *Acta Otolaryngol (Stockh)* 1976; 82: 437– 439.

16. DeSanto LW. T3 glottic cancer: options and consequences of the options. *Laryngoscope* 1984; 94: 1311–1315.

17. Lundgren JA, Gilbert RW, van Nostrand AW *et al*. T3N0M0 glottic carcinoma – a failure analysis. *Clin Otolaryngol* 1988; 1: 455–465.

18. Hong WK, Bromer R. Chemotherapy in head and neck cancer. *N Engl J Med* 1983; 308: 75–79.

19. Shirinian MH, Weber R, Lippman SM *et al*. Laryngeal preservation by induction chemotherapy plus radiotherapy in locally advanced head and neck cancer: The M.D. Anderson Cancer Center experience. *Head Neck* 1994; 16: 39–44.

20. The Department of Veterans Affairs Laryngeal Cancer Study Group. Induction chemotherapy plus radiation compared with surgery plus radiation in patients with advanced laryngeal cancer. *N Engl J Med* 1991; 324: 1685–1690.

CHAPTER four

Complications of
total laryngectomy

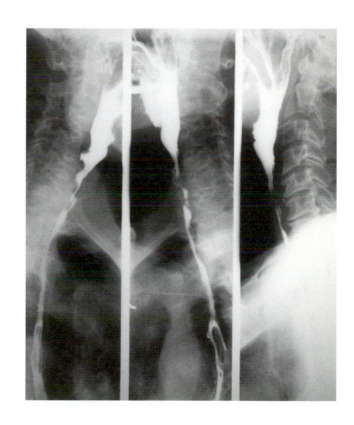

Introduction

After total laryngectomy, the patient is managed following the general principles of care following major surgical procedures. The patient's vital signs are monitored with adequate fluid and oxygen administration. Special points of note should include the maintenance of a clean tracheostomy with appropriate humidification of the air. Wound care should include the monitoring of the viability of the neck flaps and adequate functioning of the wound drains.

The common problems that might follow total laryngectomy can be grouped into early and late complications. The former include bleeding, haematoma formation, infection, dehiscence of the neck wound and pharyngocutaneous fistula. Late complications are hypothyroidism with or without hypocalcaemia, tracheostomal stenosis and stricture of the neopharynx.

Early complications

Bleeding and haematoma formation are related to poor intraoperative haemostasis and are easily recognized when the wound drain is functioning properly. A small amount of oozing from the wound area is not unexpected, and this usually abates after application of a moderate amount of pressure. When bleeding continues, or when the haematoma increases and the drain is not functioning properly, then the patient should be returned to the operating theatre for evacuation of the blood clot and meticulous haemostasis.

Primary wound dehiscence is uncommon, as a transverse incision for removal of the larynx should not give rise to any tension on closing the neck wound. Necrosis of the skin flap is infrequently seen, despite large doses of radiation being given before surgery in many patients. Patients suffering from systemic disease such as diabetes mellitus, or those taking steroids, should be monitored with particular care. Wound dehiscence and flap ischaemia may occur when too thin a skin flap has been raised, or when there is underlying infection.

Neck wound infection is relatively uncommon in patients undergoing total laryngectomy, despite previous radiotherapy in many patients. The vascularity of neck tissues and the administration of appropriate antibiotics before and during surgery helps to prevent infection. Whenever features of sepsis develop in the neck after total laryngectomy, an underlying cause such as a pharyngeal fistula should be suspected. Prompt identification of any leakage and drainage contributes to a short convalescence (Table 4.1).

Pharyngocutaneous fistula

Diagnosis

The incidence of fistula formation is higher in patients who have received large doses of radiation therapy before surgery [1]. In patients with compromised nutritional status, decreased healing ability of the pharyngeal wall may be responsible for the development of pharyngocutaneous fistula. A positive resection margin has also been identified as another factor leading to fistula [2], which once developed is associated with a poor prognosis.

Pharyngocutaneous fistulation (Box 4.1) may occur from 1–4 weeks after total laryngectomy. Early dehiscence of the pharyngeal closure usually presents as erythema and oedema around the wound. It is difficult to confirm the diagnosis of minor leakage of the neopharynx, especially in the early postoperative period because of the surrounding tissue oedema. Clinically, it may appear as a wound infection that does not respond to conservative treatment. Under these circumstances, the presence of dehiscence of the pharyngeal closure should be suspected.

A small pharyngeal leak into the surrounding tissue may be confirmed by imaging studies involving the swallow of contrast medium (Fig. 4.1). Fistulation from the pharynx to skin is suspected when saliva is seen on

Table 4.1 *Early complications after total laryngectomy, their prevention and management*

Complications	Prevention	Management
Bleeding with haematoma formation	Haemostasis during operation	Evacuation of clot and haemostasis in operating theatre
Wound infection	Preoperative antibiotics, wound irrigation	Wound culture, intravenous antibiotics
Wound dehiscence	Flap elevation of appropriate thickness	Debridement and rule out underlying fistula
Pharyngocutaneous fistula	Tensionless closure of neopharynx	Early drainage or exteriorization

the skin surface. Its presence can be confirmed by a methylene blue swallowing test.

A large fistula is usually evident clinically as there may be significant tissue necrosis beneath the skin with saliva discharging through the neck wound (Fig. 4.2). When drainage is inadequate, the contained infection may lead to septicaemia or erosion of surrounding vessels, and produce severe haemorrhage.

Management

Once the presence of pharyngeal mucosal dehiscence is suspected, drainage should be carried out. Saliva, when allowed to accumulate in the surrounding soft tissues, will lead to abscess formation and this may cause significant necrosis especially in the irradiated neck. Once formed, an abscess has a tendency to drain through a weaker point in the wound, which is the midline. The subsequently formed fistula will thus discharge directly opposite the terminal tracheostomy, leading to persistent aspiration that is very difficult to manage. Once a pharyngeal leakage is suspected, early drainage of the wound releases tissue tension and avoids the formation of a large fistula. The site chosen for drainage also diverts the route of drainage from the fistula tract. Ideally, the cutaneous opening of the fistula should be directed towards the lateral aspect of the neck, away from the terminal tracheostomy.

For an established small fistula, or a sinus tract that ends in nearby tissues with minimal necrosis, conservative management may be administered. Adequate nutrition of the patient is provided via a feeding tube. With proper wound care, a small fistula or sinus usually heals within

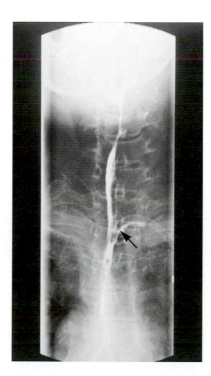

Figure 4.1 Barium swallow, the contrast outlining a small leakage of a pharyngeal closure (arrow).

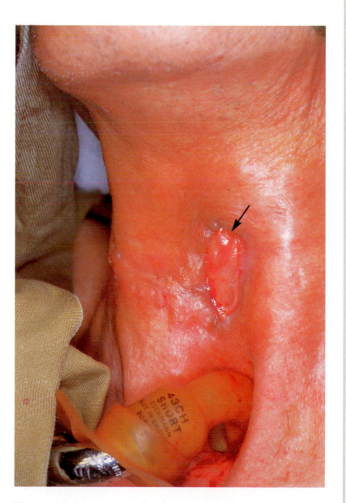

Figure 4.2 Severe wound infection revealing an underlying dehiscence of the pharyngeal closure with exposed mucosa (arrow).

2–3 weeks, depending on the general condition of the patient and whether previous radiotherapy has been given. A persistent fistula signifies either the presence of distal obstruction such as stenosis of the pharynx or recurrent tumour.

When a patient suffers from major dehiscence of the pharyngeal repair, adequate drainage of the fistula should be established. Progress is reflected by the fact that discharge from the fistula is localized and the surrounding tissue responses are minimal. Unless this is established quickly, then a full exploration of the wound should be carried out as soon as possible to reduce adjacent tissue destruction, and to avoid erosion of the great vessels and their branches.

A pharyngeal leak should be converted into a pharyngostoma by suturing the pharyngeal mucosa to the surrounding skin, thus preventing spillage of saliva into subcutaneous tissues. Following construction of this controlled pharyngostoma, the saliva may be drained locally and collected into an adhesive bag. Without further contamination, infection will subside and the pharyngostoma may be repaired at a secondary stage.

Surgical repair of a controlled pharyngostoma should be performed with non-irradiated tissue, preferably a pedicled myocutaneous flap from the chest wall. The pectoralis major myocutaneous flap is employed more frequently than the latissimus dorsi myocutaneous flap as the procedure can be carried out with the patient in the supine position alone (Fig. 4.3).

For closure of the fistula, the edge of the pharyngostoma should be fashioned afresh and the pectoralis major myocutaneous flap raised from the side closer to the pharyngostoma. The skin island of the flap is inset to close the fistula with the cutaneous component facing inwards (Fig. 4.4). As the myocutaneous muscle has significant bulk, it is not easy to close the overlying neck skin primarily once the flap is in place. A split-thickness skin graft may then be employed to cover the muscle externally. As this is on intact muscle, it does not contract, and the neck tissues feel pliable and soft (Fig. 4.5).

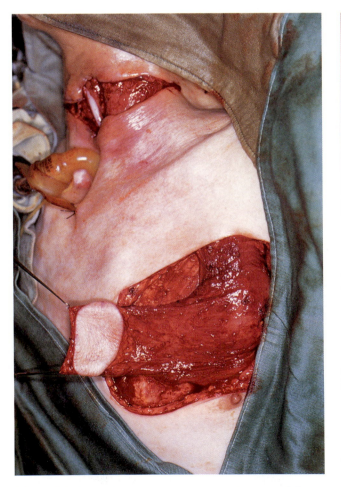

Figure 4.3 Pectoralis major myocutaneous flap raised from the chest wall for closure of the pharyngocutaneous fistula.

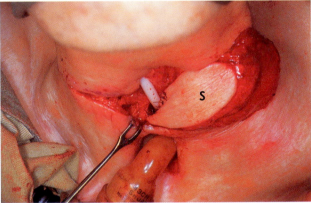

Figure 4.4 Skin island (S) over the pectoralis major muscle is turned inwards for closure of the pharyngocutaneous fistula.

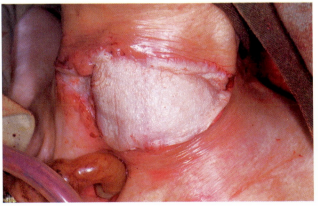

Figure 4.5 Split-thickness skin graft is laid over the muscle bulk of the pectoralis major myocutaneous flap.

Table 4.2 *Late complications after total laryngectomy, their prevention and management*

Complications	Prevention	Management
Hypothyroidism ± hypocalcaemia	Preservation of thyroid and parathyroid gland whenever possible	Thyroxine, calcium and vitamin D administration whenever indicated
Tracheostomal stenosis	Cruciate skin incision for tracheostome construction	Tracheostomy tube or revision of tracheostome. Dilatation and stent with stomal button ± revision
Stricture of the neopharynx	Ensure adequate width of the pharyngeal remnant before primary closure	Resection and reconstruction of the neopharynx if indicated

Late complications

Conditions which may affect the patients' well-being are stenosis of the terminal tracheostomy, stricture formation of the neopharynx and hypothyroidism with or without hypocalcaemia (Table 4.2).

Endocrine dysfunction

Hypoparathyroidism

When total thyroidectomy is carried out with the total laryngectomy for tumour clearance, attempts should be made to preserve the parathyroid glands. Sometimes this is not feasible, either because of macroscopic tumour extension or because there are enlarged lymph nodes in the vicinity, and any conservative form of surgical procedure may jeopardize tumour clearance.

When all the parathyroid glands have been removed, the patient develops hypocalcaemia during the early postoperative period. Clinical symptoms of cramps and circumoral parasthesia, together with signs of hypo-

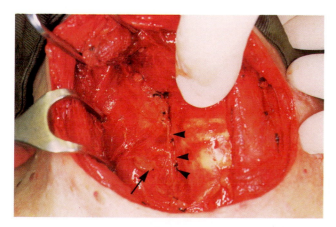

Figure 4.6 One parathyroid gland (arrow) identified close to the recurrent laryngeal nerve (arrowheads).

calcaemia may be present on the second or the third postoperative day. Intravenous calcium replacement is mandatory. When enteric feeding is started either perorally or via a nasogastric tube, calcium supplements and calciferol should be administered. The dosage should be adjusted accordingly to maintain an adequate serum calcium level and render the patient asymptomatic.

Occasionally, even when one or two parathyroid glands are preserved (Fig. 4.6), their blood supply may not be adequate and, in conjunction with postoperative radiotherapy, this may also lead to hypocalcaemia. The onset is usually insidious and symptoms of low serum calcium may appear months or years after primary surgery. Adequate serum levels of calcium can usually be maintained with peroral replacement.

Hypothyroidism

When total thyroidectomy has been carried out with total laryngectomy, then thyroxine replacement should be given during the postoperative period. If the initial resection included hemithyroidectomy, then adequate thyroid function can usually be maintained. However, if postoperative radiotherapy has been given, then on occasion thyroid function may gradually decrease. Thyroid function tests should be carried out at regular intervals during the follow-up period, and thyroid replacement therapy (thyroxine) should be given when indicated.

Stenosis of the terminal tracheostomy

Aetiology

Stenosis of a terminal tracheostomy may lead to inconvenience for the patient. It may cause difficulties in sputum removal and may limit the pulmonary capacity of the patient. Factors which cause stenosis of the terminal tracheostomy have been subjected to multivariate analysis. Female sex and infection around the tracheostomy have been identified as being of independent prognostic value [3]. The absolute tracheal diameter is smaller in females, and scar formation increases following infection. It has also been recognized that insertion of a tracheo-oesophageal voice prosthesis may lead to an increased incidence of stomal stenosis. This is most likely related to the fact that repeated insertion of the prosthesis causes some infection and subsequently scar formation (Fig. 4.7).

Management

When the size of the tracheostomy is reduced to less than 1 cm in diameter, then symptoms often occur (Fig. 4.8). Recurrence of tumour should be ruled out in all patients who develop stomal stenosis. For those patients who have a higher chance of developing this complication, a stomal button placed in the terminal tracheostomy soon after operation might decrease the likelihood of stenosis (Fig. 4.9). The button, however, interferes with the use of the tracheo-oesophageal voice prosthesis. Furthermore, the additional pressure related to the button could itself induce scar formation; thus, buttons should be used with great care in selected patients. It is better to prevent formation of the tracheostomy stenosis by transecting the

trachea obliquely when the length of tracheal remnant is adequate, or by fashioning an interdigitating suture line at the tracheocutaneous junction as described.

For established stenosis of the terminal trachea, revision of the terminal tracheostomy is performed under general anaesthesia if the patient's condition permits. Adequate mobilization of the trachea is carried out and, together with precise dissection and apposition of tissues, this can reduce the risk of recurrent stenosis. When general anaesthesia is considered inadvisable, surgery may be performed under local anaesthesia. With general anaesthesia, ventilation of the patient should be maintained with a high-frequency jet. The size of the jet is small and does not interfere with apposition of the tracheocutaneous suture line (Fig. 4.10).

The edge of the stenosis is excised and the wound edges are refashioned. Skin incisions are positioned as four radiating lines from the central trachea. In this way, four skin flaps are raised and lifted with underlying soft tissues. This is similar to the method described for primary construction of the terminal tracheostomy [4].

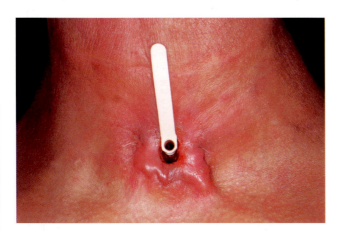

Figure 4.7 The presence of the voice prosthesis induces excessive scarring which leads to tracheostomal stenosis.

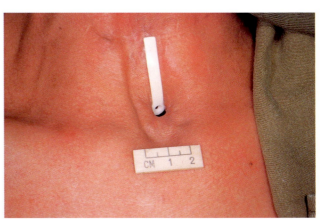

Figure 4.8 The tracheostomy is contracted to less than 1 cm in diameter, and this leads to symptoms.

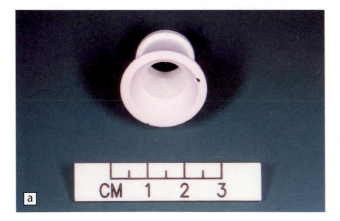

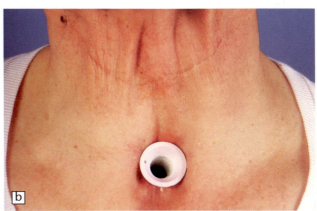

Figure 4.9 (a) Photograph of a stomal button. (b) The stomal button stents a narrow terminal tracheostomy.

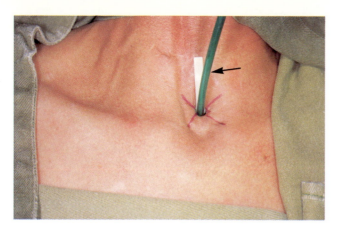

Figure 4.10 Markings for the incisions for revision of tracheostomal stenosis. The ventilation of the patient is achieved by a high-frequency jet ventilation catheter (arrow).

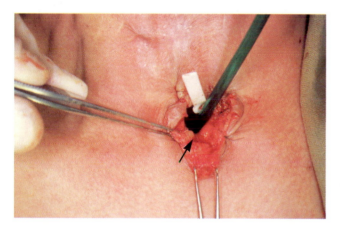

Figure 4.11 The three cutaneous flaps raised and inset into the three vertical slits placed along the vertical axis of the terminal trachea after excision of the stenotic segment (arrow).

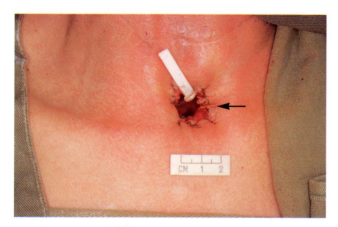

Figure 4.12 Revised tracheostomy completed, showing the wavy mucocutaneous suture line (arrow).

The tracheal stump is mobilized as far as possible, keeping close to the tracheal wall without damaging its blood supply. The stenotic ring which usually is shorter than 0.5 cm is excised, after which vertical slits 1 cm in length are made on the four walls of the trachea. The four skin flaps can then be inset into the corresponding gaps created by splitting the tracheal walls and tracheocutaneous apposition achieved with interrupted sutures (Fig. 4.11). The final suture line has a wave form rather than being circular in shape, and this reduces the incidence of future tracheostomal stenosis (Fig. 4.12).

Stricture of the neopharynx

It has been shown that when neopharynx is reconstructed with primary closure, then the pharyngeal remnant should be more than 3 cm wide to allow the patient to restore normal swallowing function [5]. In some patients, despite an apparently adequate pharyngeal lumen at the time of surgery, with the passage of time and radiotherapy stricture formation may manifest as dysphagia several years after the initial procedure. The patient usually complains of progressive dysphagia and sometimes can tolerate only a fluid diet. The diagnosis is usually suspected from the clinical features, and the degree of stenosis and length of the stricture may be confirmed with contrast image studies (Fig. 4.13). These investigations and an

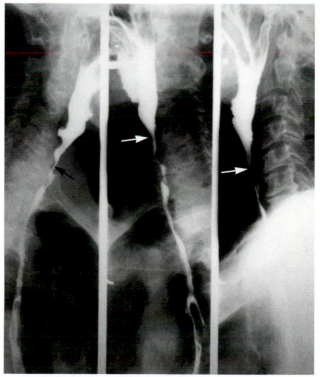

Figure 4.13 Barium swallow showing stricture of the neopharynx (arrow).

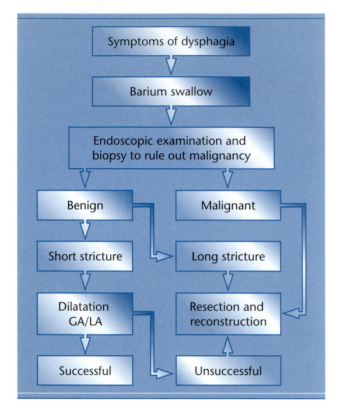

Figure 4.14 Management of neopharyngeal stricture. GA/LA, general anaesthesia/local anaesthesia.

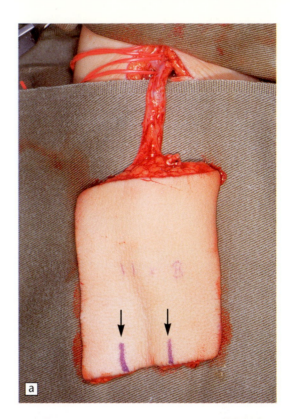

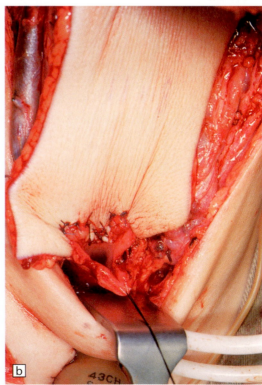

Figure 4.15 (a) Free radial forearm flap skin tubed to replace the resected strictured segment of the neopharynx. The skin was incised to allow interdigitating suturing at the mucocutaneous junction (arrows). (b) The skin island insetted to form a tube with interdigitating mucocutaneous suture line.

endoscopic examination are mandatory to rule out a second primary tumour in the oesophagus, or the presence of recurrent tumour in the neopharynx.

Management (see Fig. 4.14)

If the pharyngeal stricture is confirmed to be benign in nature, it can usually be managed conservatively with dilatation using long elastic bougies. When the stricture is not tight, the patient can be dilated under local anaesthesia in the outpatient clinic. For patients with a tight and small stricture, then the initial dilatation should be carried out under general anaesthesia. The dilatation should be gentle so as not to create false tracts or produce bleeding. With too much tissue trauma, the formation of reparative fibrosis will lead to even more stenosis. When a reasonable-sized lumen is obtained with the initial dilatation, then subsequent maintenance dilatation is performed in the outpatient clinic.

For the patient who develops a long stricture or when dilatation is not successful, surgical treatment should be offered to relieve dysphagia. It is not advisable to split the neopharynx and use a myocutaneous patch to augment the circumference of the pharyngeal wall. As a result of stricture formation, the lumen is usually so narrow that after splitting there is virtually no pharyngeal mucosa left. It is much easier to perform a circumferential pharyngectomy and to replace the entire segment of the neopharynx from the tongue base to the oesophagus.

A microvascular free jejunal graft is the option of choice for reconstruction of circumferential pharyngeal defect [6]. A free radial forearm flap can also be sutured in such a way as to form a tubular skin tube for reconstruction (Fig. 4.15). The free jejunal graft is superior in that both upper and lower anastomoses are circular, and there is no 'T' junction along the suture lines. Mucosa-to-mucosa suturing of the jejunum has a lesser chance of stricture formation at the anastomotic site. The production of mucus in the jejunum also contributes to smooth swallowing. The use of free jejunum requires the expertise of microvascular anastomosis and recipient vessels in the neck to provide a blood supply (Fig. 4.16). If such expertise is not available, or when there are no suitable vessels in the neck for vascular anastomosis, then the tubed pectoralis major myocutaneous flap can be used for reconstruction of a

circumferential pharyngeal defect. Under these circumstances, suturing of the skin to the mucosa should be performed in an interdigitating fashion to prevent stenosis at the anastomotic site [7] (Figs 4.17, 4.18). The incidence of leakage is higher with the tubed pectoralis major myocutaneous flap (Fig. 4.19) when compared with free flaps, and a longer convalescent period is to be expected.

Summary

Complications of total laryngectomy can be grouped into early and late phases. Pharyngocutaneous fistula belongs to the former group. When this condition is detected early, prompt treatment may prevent the formation of serious sequelae. Surgical closure is indicated when the fistula is of significant size and fails to respond to conservative treatment. Tissue from outside the radiation field is necessary for proper repair of fistula.

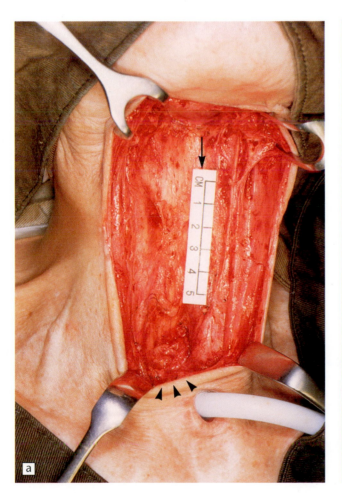
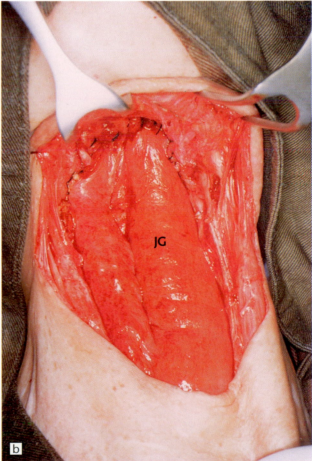

Figure 4.16 (a) Segmental defect created after circumferential pharyngectomy. Oropharyngeal opening (arrow), oesophageal opening (arrow heads). (b) Free jejunal graft (JG) used to reconstruct the defect created after circumferential pharyngectomy.

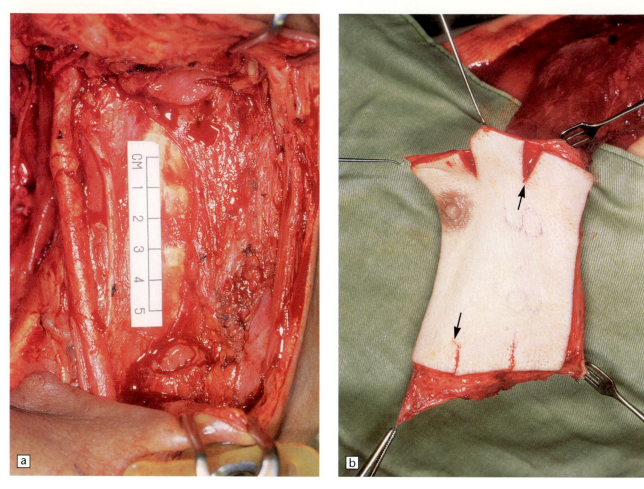

Figure 4.17 (a) Pharyngeal defect after circumferential pharyngectomy. (b) Incision over the skin island of the pectoralis major myocutaneous flap to allow the construction of a non-circular mucocutaneous suture line (arrows).

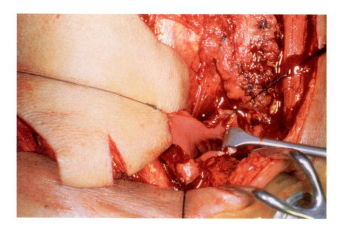

Figure 4.18 The interdigitation suturing of the mucosal and cutaneous flaps at the anastomosis.

Late complications include endocrine problems, stenosis of the terminal tracheostomy and stricture of the neopharynx. Replacement therapy is usually adequate for the endocrine dysfunction, while revision of the terminal tracheostomy with a zigzag mucocutaneous suture line is efficient in preventing future stenosis.

For stricture of the neopharynx, recurrent tumour must first be excluded, and when the narrowing is not severe, intermittent dilatation with bougies usually solves the problem. When the stricture is too tight or when dilatation fails, then resection of the entire pharyngeal segment is necessary. The circumferential pharyngeal defect can be replaced with microvascular free jejunal graft or a tubed pedicled myocutaneous flap.

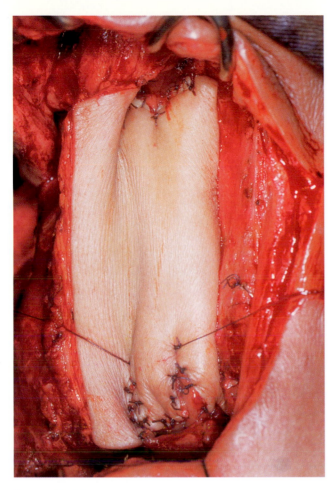

Figure 4.19 The skin island of pectoralis major muscle formed into a tube.

References

1. Wei WI, Lam KH, Wong J, Ong GB. Pharyngocutaneous fistula complicating total laryngectomy. *Aust NZ J Surg* 1980; 50: 366–369.

2. Shemen LJ, Spiro RH. Complications following laryngectomy. *Head Neck Surg* 1986; 8: 185–191.

3. Kuo M, Ho CM, Wei WI, Lam KH. Tracheostomal stenosis after total laryngectomy: an analysis of predisposing clinical factors. *Laryngoscope* 1994; 104: 59–63.

4. Lam KH, Wei WI, Wong J, Ong GB. Tracheostome construction during laryngectomy – a method to prevent stenosis. *Laryngoscope* 1983; 93: 212–215.

5. Hui Y, Wei WI, Yuen PW *et al*. Primary closure of pharyngeal remnant after total laryngectomy and partial pharyngectomy: how much residual mucosa is sufficient. *Laryngoscope* 1996; 106: 490–494.

6. de Vries EJ, Myers EN, Johnson JT *et al*. Jejunal interposition for repair of stricture or fistula after laryngectomy. *Ann Otol Rhinol Laryngol* 1990; 99: 496–498.

7. Lam KH, Wei WI, Lau WF. Avoiding stenosis in the tubed greater pectoral flap in pharyngeal repair. *Arch Otolaryngol Head Neck Surg* 1987; 113: 428–431.

CHAPTER five

Radiotherapy for
laryngeal cancer

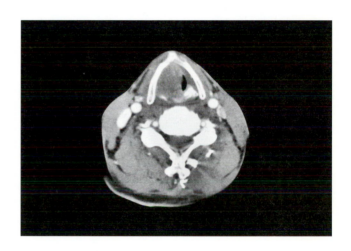

Rationale of radical primary radiotherapy, preoperative and postoperative radiotherapy

In the treatment of laryngeal cancer, the aims are to obtain optimal cure rates with the best functional results. The choice of treatment (Box 5.1) depends on the local control rate, the chance of successful salvage treatment when the primary treatment fails, the chance of saving the laryngeal voice, and the quality of the voice so saved. The availability of expertise in both surgery and radiotherapy are also important determinants of choice in treatment.

The factors that influence tumour control after radiotherapy relate to the size of the tumour: larger tumours require higher doses of radiation, treatment of a larger volume, and the inclusion of more normal structures. The inclusion of larger volume and more normal structures will in turn increase the chance of complications, and result in an inferior voice. Because of these limitations set by the normal tissue, the chance of tumour control using radiotherapy alone is often compromised in the case of advanced lesions.

For small laryngeal tumours, the chance of tumour control with radiotherapy is good, as is the quality of voice preserved [1,2]. For larger laryngeal tumours, in order to achieve optimal tumour control, a combination of surgery and radiotherapy is usually adopted (Table 5.1). In theory, it is possible to combine surgery and radiotherapy in two different sequences. From the consideration of radiobiology (Table 5.2), preoperative radiotherapy

Table 5.1 *Recommended treatment for glottic and supraglottic cancers by stage*

Tumour stage	Treatment
T1	Surgery or radiotherapy
T2	Surgery or radiotherapy for glottic cancers, surgery plus postoperative radiotherapy for supraglottic cancers
T3 or T4	Surgery plus postoperative radiotherapy

has the advantage of well-oxygenated tissue in the target volume (hypoxia is a potent cause of radioresistance), and the preoperative radiation given will decrease the viability of the tumour cells and hence the chance of spread of tumour by local seeding and blood-borne spread during surgery. However, in practice surgery is usually attempted first, followed by postoperative radiotherapy. This is because preoperative radiotherapy will increase postoperative surgical complications, and there is a significant chance of patients defaulting from surgery after a partial response of tumour has been achieved with preoperative radiotherapy.

In the management of supraglottic cancers with radical radiotherapy, the treatment of neck nodes must be given special consideration because of the propensity of lymph node spread.

Radiation techniques

Telecobalt units or linear accelerators producing 4–6 MeV photons are ideal for treating the subcutaneous tissues while sparing the overlying skin. Treatment will usually begin with parallel lateral opposing cervical fields, the size of which is determined by the size and extent of the primary tumour (information is obtained from endoscopic examination and imaging), as well as the extent and potential extension of nodal involvement (Box 5.2).

For patients who require large fields that cover the spinal cord, after 40–45 Gy (when the spinal cord tolerance has been reached) the lateral opposing cervical fields

Box 5.1 *Factors influencing choice of treatment for laryngeal cancers*

- Size of tumour (T stage)
- Chance of preserving laryngeal voice and its quality
- Availability of expertise in surgery and radiotherapy
- Preference of patient
- General poor health of patient may exclude surgery

Table 5.2 *Advantages and disadvantages of preoperative radiotherapy*

Advantages	Disadvantages
Well-oxygenated tumour, more sensitive to radiotherapy	Increased postoperative surgical complications
Decrease viability of tumour cells and hence chance of spread during surgery	Patient default planned surgery after partial response of tumour to radiotherapy

must be reduced to protect the spinal cord (Table 5.3). The posterior limit of field is reduced to the posterior one-third of the vertebral body, and the posterior neck is treated with electron beams, aiming at total dose of 55–70 Gy depending on the size of the nodal disease. If the tumour is not extensive, the field may be further reduced after 55–60 Gy to avoid the oropharynx and upper cervical oesophagus. The total dose to the primary tumour should be 66–70 Gy.

For the posterior neck treatment using electron beams, the depth of tissue to be treated may be adjusted by choosing the energy of the electron beam. The thickness of tissue to be treated, and the depth of spinal cord which needs to be protected, are best assessed with computed tomography (CT) scanning.

Except for small glottic tumours without neck node involvement (when the risk of occult neck node involvement is small), a matching lower anterior cervical field is used from the beginning to cover the lower one-third of cervical lymphatics, the apices of the lung being shielded below the clavicles. A midline shield is required after 45 Gy to protect the spinal cord. The total dose to be given with this field is determined by the extent of nodal involvement.

When a matching lower anterior cervical field is used, a 1-cm shield should be added to the posterio-inferior corner of the lateral opposing cervical fields to avoid beam overlap at the spinal cord.

To ensure reproducibility of treatment position, the accuracy of the marks required to direct the beams, and to avoid putting the marks on a patient's skin, a mould is required for all cases. This is usually done with the patient in the supine position and, under fluoroscopy screening, using a simulator to ensure that the alignment of the cervical spine is straight in the anteroposterior and lateral directions. This facilitates shielding of the spinal cord from the lateral opposing beams in the second phase of the treatment (Box 5.3). The clinically palpable nodes are marked out on the skin with radio-opaque wire so that they may be localized on the simulator check film. There is an option of having a set of CT scans repeated in the treatment position with the mould; these scans can be used for localization of tumour as well as three-dimensional computation of dose distribution. Customized compensators may be required to achieve homogeneity of dose because the thickness of the target volume often varies considerably between the upper part of the beam and the lower cervical region.

A final verification of accuracy is performed at the treatment machine, with check films taken to ensure that the coverage of the radiation fields is as planned.

Supraglottic tumours

There is high risk of nodal involvement, and data from elective neck dissections indicate an approximately 30%

Table 5.3 *Small-field versus large-field irradiation*

	Small-field	Large-field
Indications	For early primary tumour without neck node involvement, and low risk of occult nodal involvement	For advanced primary tumour or nodal involvement, or with high risk of occult nodal involvement
Anatomical considerations	Can be adequately covered with lateral opposing fields	In order to cover the spinoaccessory chain of neck nodes, the spinal cord will be included in the treatment volume with lateral opposing fields. In order to cover the lower cervical lymphatics and upper oesophagus, a matching lower anterior cervical field is required
Need to change treatment field set-up	No need as spinal cord is outside of treatment volume	Need to reduce posterior border of lateral opposing fields after 45 Gy in order to protect spinal cord, posterior neck treatment to be continued with electron beam
Side effects	Less acute and late side effects	More acute and late side effects

- Patient lying supine, position of head determined under fluoroscopic screening to ensure cervical spine is straight
- Cast of head and neck region made in this position
- Option 1 of taking a set of CT scans with this cast for localizing tumour
- Option 2 of taking X-radiograph with simulator for localizing tumour
- Determine the margins required and size of radiation field
- Computation of dose and use of beam compensators if necessary
- Verification by taking check films with treatment machine

Box 5.4 *Additional factors affecting radiotherapy for laryngeal cancers*

- 30% chance of occult nodal involvement in clinical N0 disease for supraglottic cancers
- Pre-epiglottic extension of tumour is an area prone to underdosing
- Tracheostoma (for airway obstruction or after laryngectomy) is a common site of recurrence

Box 5.5 *Field arrangement for supraglottic cancers*

- 2–3 cm margin for primary tumour and involved nodes for the first 60 Gy
- Prophylactic neck treatment with superior field margin to cover tip of mastoid for all cases
- Prophylactic neck treatment of lower cervical lymphatics for patients with neck node involvement, using matching lower anterior cervical field

chance of occult nodal involvement in clinical N0 disease. Nodal relapse is also a common cause of failure (Box 5.4).

For early disease, the control rate is comparable with that achieved by surgery, but there is the additional advantage of giving bilateral prophylactic neck irradiation, which is simple and has few side effects. For similar staged lesions, there is no difference in local control with radiotherapy for tumours involving different subsites.

For more advanced disease, the extent of pre-epiglottic involvement and tumour bulk are important prognostic factors, in addition to vocal cord invasion.

Radiotherapy technique

The usual treatment consists of two lateral opposing fields for the primary site and the neck lymphatics, with a separate anterior field for the lower neck. A margin of 2–3 cm should be allowed for the primary tumour and positive nodes, while the upper cervical lymphatics should always be covered by extending the upper margin of field to cover the tip of mastoid (Box 5.5). For patients with tracheostomy, the stoma must be included in the treatment volume. The spinal cord dose should be limited to 45 Gy. When this spinal cord dose is reached,

the posterior border of the lateral opposing fields will be brought forward to protect the spinal cord. The lateral opposing treatment fields may be further reduced in size to allow a margin of 1.5 cm for the primary tumour and positive nodes after 60 Gy has been given. For T1 and T2 lesions, a tumour dose of 65–68 Gy should be aimed for. For more advanced diseases, 70 Gy or more is required.

Treatment in the posterior neck is to be continued with electron beams of appropriate energy, aiming at a total dose of 55–70 Gy depending on the size of nodal disease. The depth of tissue to be treated may be adjusted by choosing the energy of the electron beam. The thickness of tissue to be treated, and the depth of spinal cord which needs to be protected, are best assessed from CT scans.

The anterior tapering contour of the neck has two implications on radiotherapy: (i) dose homogeneity should be maintained using tissue compensators; and (ii) the photon energy should not be higher than 6 MV in order to avoid underdosing the tissue in the anterior tapering part of neck due to lack of tissue overlaying the tumour. Special attention to this area is important when the tumour involves the lower end of the epiglottis, as this is the site of pre-epiglottic extension of tumour. In thin patients, the prominence of the thyroid cartilage requires bolus up to prevent underdosing of the pre-epiglottic space.

Treatment of the lower cervical lymphatics is required in patients with neck node involvement. Initially using a matching lower anterior cervical field, the apices of the lung are shielded below the clavicles. A midline shield is required after 45 Gy to protect the spinal cord. The total dose to be given with this field is determined by the extent of nodal involvement. Elective neck irradiation is indicated for N0 disease because of the high risk of occult nodal involvement [3].

When a matching lower anterior cervical field is used, a 1-cm shield should be added to the posterio-inferior corner of the lateral opposing cervical fields in order to avoid beam overlap at the spinal cord.

Recent studies have reported better results with hyperfractionation radiotherapy [4], but this is probably required only for advanced disease. In hyperfractionation radiotherapy (Box 5.6), more than one fractional treatment is given per day, with the dose being smaller than a conventional fractional dose of 2 Gy; the aim is to achieve a shorter overall treatment time. This in turn will partially circumvent the accelerated growth of tumour that is triggered by radiotherapy and which is an important cause of treatment failure. As the late complications of radiotherapy (e.g. radiochondronecrosis of the larynx) are a function of the fractional dose, the smaller fractional dose used in hyperfractionation radiotherapy will compensate for the higher total dose to be given. However, the acute side effects (mainly in the form of mucositis), which depend on the total dose to be given and are the result of the balance of accelerated normal tissue recovery versus cell killing induced by radiation, will be exaggerated. The end result of hyperfractionation radiotherapy will be an improvement in tumour control, but accompanied by exaggerated acute reactions.

Using radiotherapy alone, the local control for T1, T2, T3 and T4 supraglottic tumours is reported as 100%, 81%, 61% and 33%, respectively [5,6]. Local control for T2 and T3 supraglottic tumours with total laryngectomy plus postoperative radiotherapy were 88% and 64%, respectively [7].

Glottic tumours

For in-situ lesions, radiotherapy provides similar control as does stripping of the vocal cords, and a better quality of voice. Although surgical treatment allows detailed examination of the specimen while radiotherapy does not (as control of the tumour is the primary aim), there is little practical difference between the two regimes. Nonetheless, early treatment with radiotherapy is advised as it is difficult to exclude invasion, and disease will progress to invasion in most patients. Thus, most patients would eventually require this treatment – which has few side effects.

For T1 tumours, 83–93% local control is achieved with radiotherapy [8,9], while for T2 tumours, 67–88% local control is achieved [10,11]. Impairment of the mobility of the vocal cords, indicating infiltration by tumour, is associated with poorer control [12]. Involvement of the anterior commissure is another potential adverse prognostic factor, because of the associated pre-epiglottic extension of tumour. Although the adverse prognostic value of anterior commissure involvement has not been substantiated [13], this is considered to be important by oncologists. The current treatment technique has already taken this factor into consideration.

Radiotherapy technique

The normal treatment consists of two lateral opposing fields to cover the primary site. For early tumours, a field size of 5 × 5 cm to 6 × 6 cm is usually required. With fields centred on the vocal cords, the superior border of fields should cover the thyroid notch, the inferior border should cover the cricoid cartilage, the anterior border should adequately cover the skin over the thyroid eminence (pre-epiglottic space), and the posterior border should cover the anterior part of the posterior pharyngeal wall (Box 5.7). A total tumour dose of 66 Gy is required.

Larger fields will be required for more extensive tumours [14] and when there is neck node involvement. In these cases, spinal cord protection will be achieved with a reduction in field size after 45 Gy is reached, and treatment of the posterior neck is continued with electron beam.

For glottic cancers, elective radiotherapy for the drainage lymphatics using a pair of larger lateral opposing cervical fields is not required. Covering those adjacent lymphatics which would have been covered by fields intended for the primary tumour would be adequate.

Matching the lower anterior cervical field is usually not required in primary radiotherapy for glottic cancers, as the chance of moderate to extensive nodal involvement is small.

The anterior tapering contour of neck has the same implications as for radiotherapy of supraglottic cancers. Thus, dose homogeneity should be maintained using tissue compensators, and the photon beam energy should not be higher than 6 MV in order to avoid underdosing the anterior tapering tip of the neck. This is especially important when there is involvement of the anterior commissure, as this is the site of pre-epiglottic extension of tumour. In thin patients, the prominence of the thyroid cartilage requires bolus up in order to prevent underdosing the pre-epiglottic space.

Organ preservation using combined induction chemotherapy and radiotherapy

For patients with stage III and IV glottic cancers, the usual scheme of organ preservation treatment consists of two courses of induction chemotherapy using cisplatin and 5-fluorouracil, those patients showing partial or better response will generally proceed to a third cycle followed by radiotherapy. Those patients showing less response or who relapse will undergo laryngectomy. With such treatment, the Veterans Affairs Laryngeal Study Group reported laryngeal preservation in 64% of patients, the treatment being well tolerated [15] (Box 5.8). An update of results from this study showed that long-term disease-free survival was more likely to occur in patients who achieved a complete response to induction chemotherapy; results in non-responding patients were not adversely affected when prompt salvage surgery was

given [16]. A long-term functional and quality of life study on the same group of patients showed that they were better off in terms of speech communication [17], had a better quality of life, more freedom from pain, better emotional well-being and a lower level of depression [18]. However, a study showing adverse results after induction chemotherapy has also been reported [19]. In view of the suboptimal results reported – especially in those patients with a less than complete response to chemotherapy – induction chemotherapy plus radiotherapy for organ preservation should not be offered routinely outside the protocol studies.

Postoperative radiotherapy

For T3 glottic or T2/T3 supraglottic cancers, a combination of surgery and radiotherapy provides better control than either radiotherapy or surgery alone. By combining total laryngectomy and postoperative radiotherapy, 75% local-regional control was achieved for T3 glottic cancer [20]. Local control for T2 and T3 supraglottic tumours with total laryngectomy plus postoperative radiotherapy was 88% and 64%, respectively [7].

Ideally, the patients should be assessed by both surgeons and radiation oncologists before surgery (Box 5.9), so that the initial extent of disease is known to the latter group. At about one week after surgery, when the patient is fit, an assessment by the radiation oncologists should be made and preparation for radiotherapy arranged, so that treatment may be started at about 3–4 weeks after surgery. Treatment must be delayed when surgical complications occur such as delayed wound healing, but not beyond the sixth week. The assessments include surgical operative findings and pathologist's comments on the surgical specimen, in particular paying attention to the sites at risk of failure, such as tumour involvement or a close resection margin.

Treatment usually consists of large parallel lateral opposing fields to cover the sites of the original primary

Box 5.8 *Organ preservation with induction chemotherapy plus radiotherapy in glottic cancer*

- Two courses of combination chemotherapy using cisplatin and 5-fluorouracil
- A patient who has achieved partial or better response to two courses of chemotherapy will proceed to a third course of chemotherapy to be followed with radiotherapy
- A patient with a less than partial response or with recurrence will receive prompt salvage laryngectomy
- Some 64% laryngeal preservation was obtained; survival was not adversely affected. Long-term functional and quality of life study showed improvement in speech communication, better quality of life, freedom from pain, better emotional well-being and a lower level of depression
- Adverse results have also been reported from other studies, especially for those patients who achieved only partial response from induction chemotherapy. Thus, not recommended for treatment outside of protocol study

Box 5.9 *Postoperative radiotherapy*

- Assessment of patient by surgeons and radiation oncologists before surgery so that extent of tumour known to both teams
- Cast making in preparation of radiotherapy about one week after surgery
- Planning of radiotherapy taking into consideration operative findings and pathology study of surgical specimen to identify sites at risk of failure
- Start treatment 3–4 weeks after surgery

tumour and neck node, as well as the surgical field which is potentially seeded during operation. The surgical scars are marked with metallic wires so that they may be localized on the simulator check film, the purpose being to ensure that the scars are covered with radiotherapy. For supraglottic cancers, the superior margin of field should cover the tip of the mastoid in order to treat the retropharyngeal nodes. The spinal cord dose should be limited to 45 Gy. When this dose is reached, the posterior border of the lateral opposing fields are brought forward to protect the spinal cord. The target dose should be 65–68 Gy.

A separate matching lower anterior field will be required to cover the lower cervical lymphatics and the tracheostomy, which is a common site of relapse. Elective treatment of lower cervical lymphatics is necessary in patients with supraglottic cancer, and in those with glottic and neck node involvement.

Treatment in the posterior neck should be continued with electron beams of appropriate energy, aiming at a total dose of 60–68 Gy, depending on the size of the original nodal disease. The depth of tissue to be treated may be adjusted by choosing the energy of electron beam. The thickness of tissue to be treated, and the depth of spinal cord which needs to be protected, are best assessed from a CT scan.

The change in contour in this part of the body is exaggerated by surgical removal of tissue, and the use of tissue compensators to maintain dose homogeneity will be required.

Follow-up after radiotherapy

Following radiotherapy, patients should be seen every 4–6 weeks during the first year, every 2 months in the second year, every 3 months in the third year, and every 4–6 months (or even longer intervals) during subsequent years (Box 5.10).

An examination of the larynx and neck should be performed. Follow-up using fibrescopic examination

Box 5.10 *Follow-up after radiotherapy*

- Every 4–6 weeks in the first year, every 2 months in the second year, every 3 months in the third year, every 4–6 months or longer in subsequent years
- Examination of larynx (with indirect mirror examination or fibrescope) and neck nodes
- Biopsy of larynx should be avoided unless there is strong suspicion of relapse

may be required if an indirect mirror examination is not adequate. However, biopsy should be avoided unless there is strong suspicion of tumour recurrence, such as evidence of gross tumour, or associated pain. Biopsy after high-dose irradiation may precipitate necrosis which might result in laryngectomy.

In some cases, marked oedema associated with pain may be the only features of recurrence, and even repeated biopsies are returned as negative. In such patients, laryngectomy may still be required to confirm and treat recurrent disease. Before they consent to surgery, such patients must be informed that in a proportion of cases no tumour will be found in the surgical specimen, but only necrosis.

Examination of the neck after irradiation is hampered by the presence of oedema. In patients who originally had nodes larger than 3 cm, the chance of relapse is increased, and special attention must be paid to the neck examination at follow-up. Early detection of neck node relapse in patients treated with primary radiotherapy will be amenable to curative salvage with radical neck dissection.

Complications of radiotherapy

Significant acute mucositis in the pharynx included in the target volume will affect more than 95% of patients (Table 5.4), and result in pain that affects both swallowing

Table 5.4 *Acute and late side effects of radiotherapy*

Acute	Late
Mucositis resulting in pain, exacerbated by swallowing. Treatment is symptomatic, will improve spontaneously 2–3 weeks after completion of radiotherapy	Fibrosis of subcutaneous tissue and hypothyroidism. Both will be symptomatic in a small proportion of patients, and will be permanent
Skin reaction. Treatment is symptomatic, will improve spontaneously 2–3 weeks after completion of radiotherapy	Severe laryngeal oedema and osteochondronecrosis

and feeding. Symptoms usually start toward the end of the third to fourth week of radiotherapy, and will improve within 2 weeks after completion of treatment. Mucositis manifests as mucosal erythema or whitish patches. Treatment of mucositis is symptomatic with gargles and analgesics, but continued optimal feeding should be encouraged as impairment of nutrition might aggravate the condition.

An acute skin reaction in the form of erythema of the skin and slight pain will occur in many patients; treatment is again symptomatic.

Severe laryngeal oedema and osteochondronecrosis may occur, especially in patients with advanced tumour given high-dose irradiation.

Fibrosis of subcutaneous tissue is a common late reaction occurring 1–2 years after treatment; the degree of fibrosis will be exaggerated by the combination of neck dissection and postoperative irradiation.

Hypothyroidism due to irradiation of the thyroid gland occurs in a small proportion of patients; monitoring of thyroxine (T4) and thyroid-stimulating hormone (TSH) is required to detect subclinical cases.

Salvage treatment for recurrence

In patients who have relapsed after previous surgery, radiotherapy will offer a good chance of local control, provided that the relapse is detected early. The treatment technique is similar to that described for planned postoperative radiotherapy after surgery. Additional attention should be given to the localization of the recurrent tumour, the inclusion of other potential sites of relapse (which include the tracheostomy site) and the previous surgical field which are potential sites of seeding during the original operation.

Radiotherapy technique

Two lateral opposing fields are applied to the neck to include the recurrent tumour and the potential sites as described, with separate lower anterior field for lower cervical lymphatics and the tracheostomy. When the recurrent tumour is in the surgical scar, or is in the superficial subcutaneous region, these regions must be bolused up in order to ensure that there is no underdosing due to the skin-sparing effect of megavoltage radiotherapy.

The spinal cord dose should be limited to 45 Gy. When this is reached, the posterior border of the lateral opposing fields will be brought forward to protect the spinal cord, and the posterior neck treatment continued with electron beams of appropriate energy, aiming at total dose of 55–70 Gy, depending on the extent of recurrent disease in this part of the neck. The depth of tissue to be treated may be adjusted by choosing the energy of electron beam. The thickness of tissue to be treated, and the depth of spinal cord that needs to be protected, are best assessed from a CT scan.

References

1. Karim ABMF, Snow GB, Sick HTH, Njo KH. The quality of voice in patients irradiated for laryngeal carcinoma. *Cancer* 1983; 51: 47–49.

2. Harwood AR, Tierie A. Radiotherapy of early glottic cancer. *Int J Radiat Oncol Biol Phys* 1979; 5: 477–482.

3. Mendenhall WM, Million RR, Cassisi NJ. Elective neck irradiation in squamous cell carcinoma of the head and neck. *Head Neck Surg* 1980; 3: 15–20.

4. Parsons JT, Mendenhall WM, Millian RR. Twice-a-day irradiation of squamous cell carcinoma of the head and neck. *Semin Radiat Oncol* 1992; 2: 29–35.

5. Mendenhall WM, Parson JT, Stringer SP *et al*. Carcinoma of the supraglottic larynx: a basis for comparing the results of radiotherapy and surgery. *Head Neck* 1990; 12: 204–209.

6. Wang CC. Megavoltage radiation therapy for supraglottic carcinoma. *Radiology* 1973; 102: 183–186.

7. Goepfert H, Jesse RH, Fletcher GH, Hamberger A. Optimal treatment for the technically resectable squamous cell carcinoma of the supraglottic larynx. *Laryngoscope* 1975; 85: 14–32.

8. Mittal B. Rao DV, Marks JE, Perez CA. Role of radiation in the management of early vocal cord carcinoma. *Int J Radiat Oncol Biol Phys* 1983; 9: 997–1002.

9. Mendenhall WM, Parsons JT, Million RR, Fletcher GH. T1–T2 squamous cell carcinoma of the glottic larynx treated with radiation therapy: relationship of dose-fractionation factors to local control and complications. *Int J Radiat Oncol Biol Phys* 1988; 15: 1267–1273.

10. Le QT, Fu KK, Kroll S *et al*. Influence of time and fractionation on local control of T1, 2 glottic carcinoma. *Int J Radiat Oncol Biol Phys* 1997; 39: 115–126.

11. Amornmarn R, Prempree T, Viravathana T *et al*. A therapeutic approach to early vocal cord carcinoma. *Acta Radiol (Oncol)* 1985; 24: 321–325.

12. Van den Bogaert W, Rostyn F, van der Schuern E. The significance of extension and impaired mobility in cancer of the vocal cord. *Int J Radiat Oncol Biol Phys* 1983; 9: 181–184.

13. Woodhouse RJ, Quivey JM, Fu KK *et al*. Treatment of carcinoma of the vocal cords: a review of 20 years experience. *Laryngoscope* 1981; 91: 1155–1162.

14. Harwood AR, Beale FA, Cummings BJ *et al*. T2 glottic cancer: an analysis of dose-time-volume factors. *Int J Radiat Oncol Biol Phys* 1981; 7: 1501–1505.

15. The Department of Veterans Affairs Laryngeal Cancer Study Group. Induction chemotherapy plus radiation compared with surgery plus radiation in patients with advanced laryngeal cancer. *N Engl J Med* 1991; 324: 1685–1690.

16. Spaulding MB, Fischer SG, Wolf GT. Tumor response, toxicity, and survival after neoadjuvant organ-preserving chemotherapy for advanced laryngeal carcinoma. The Department of Veterans Affairs Cooperative Laryngeal Cancer Study Group. *J Clin Oncol* 1994; 12: 1592–1599.

17. Hillman RE, Walsh MJ, Wolf GT *et al*. Functional outcomes following treatment for advanced laryngeal cancer. Part I – Voice preservation in advanced laryngeal cancer. Part II – Laryngectomy rehabilitation: the state of the art in the VA System. *Ann Otol Rhinol Laryngol Suppl.* 1998; 172: 1–27.

18. Terrell JE, Fisher SG, Wolf GT. Long-term quality of life after treatment of laryngeal cancer. The Veterans Affairs Laryngeal Cancer Study Group. *Arch Otolaryngol Head Neck Surg* 1998; 124: 964–971.

19. Richard JM, Sancho-Garnier H, Pessey JJ *et al*. Randomized trial of induction chemotherapy in larynx carcinoma. *Oral Oncol* 1998; 34: 224–228.

20. Mendenhall WM, Parson JT, Stringer SP *et al*. Stage T3 squamous cell carcinoma of the glottic larynx: a comparison of laryngectomy and irradiation. *Int J Radiat Oncol Biol Phys* 1992; 23: 725–732.

CHAPTER six

Speech rehabilitation
after total laryngectomy

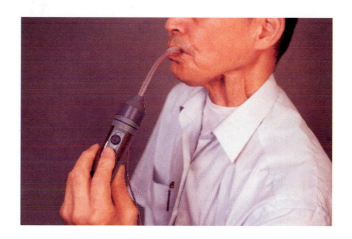

Introduction

The most frequent presenting symptom of patients suffering from carcinoma of the larynx is hoarseness, as the cancer destroys laryngeal structures or interferes with their function. The surgical treatment that is currently available sacrifices at least part of the larynx, and thus compromises vocalization which may be lost altogether when total laryngectomy is carried out for tumour eradication. The prospect of becoming voiceless after surgery is distressing and frequently contributes to delays in treatment. Patients understandably are reluctant to undergo total laryngectomy and may seek alternative treatment methods which can jeopardize prospects for cure in exchange for voice preservation. Currently, after total laryngectomy, patients can still produce intelligible speech if voice rehabilitation is successful.

Mechanism of normal speech production

The basic requirement for a normal individual to produce intelligible speech is, first, to have the ability to produce sound. Coordinated muscular movement of the pharynx, soft palate, cheek, and tongue together with positioning of teeth, patency of the nasal cavities and the degree of aeration of the paranasal sinuses, modify the sound to the characteristic speech of the individual. In a normal individual, sound is produced by controlled expiration of pulmonary air to vibrate the properly apposed vocal cords. When a patient has undergone total laryngectomy, then an alternative sound production mechanism must be established for conversion to speech (Fig. 6.1).

Currently, commonly used speech restoration modalities can be categorized into three groups, depending on the principles of sound production and whether a special device is required (Table 6.1):

- The oesophageal speech group require no additional instrument.
- Patients who have undergone tracheo-oesophageal puncture employ a prosthesis which is inserted through a surgically created fistula. This prosthesis has a one-way valve, and some models may be removed for cleansing from time to time.
- The external voice aid group, who use either an electro-larynx or a pneumatic device for sound production.

Oesophageal speech

In general, speech rehabilitation begins only when surgical wounds have healed and normal oral feeding has resumed. During the early postoperative period, the patient uses other non-verbal methods for communication, such as hand signs or writing. Some patients may try speech generated by the lips or use trapped buccal air to produce

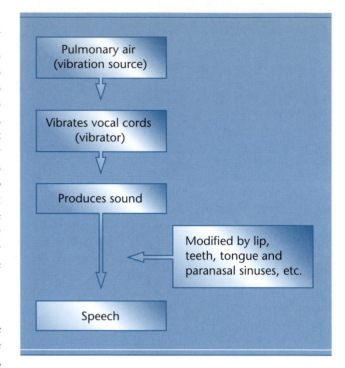

Figure 6.1 Flow chart of normal speech production.

sound and a limited form of speech. More intelligible sounds can be achieved by regurgitation of oesophageal air in order to vibrate the pharyngeal mucosa.

Patients learn to swallow, inhale or inject air into the oesophagus and when the air has reached a certain volume, it is released to vibrate the pharyngeal mucosa to produce sound. This sound is further modified appropriately by articulators such as the teeth, tongue, etc. to generate understandable speech. The volume of air that can be stored in the oesophagus may after training be 200–300 ml. This is, however, still only about one-tenth of the vital capacity of the lung; thus, the length of the sentences produced by oesophageal speech is short and these are sometimes intermittent. Intervals between sentences can be reduced when the individual has learned how to inject air into the oesophagus while speaking.

The amplitude of the voice produced by oesophageal speech is low compared with normal speech. The expiratory force of the stored air in the oesophagus is not high enough to vibrate the pharyngeal mucosa forcefully and produce a loud sound. Thus, oesophageal speech may be inaudible in a noisy environment when there is a lot of ambient sound.

In order to acquire the ability to use oesophageal speech, long periods of training are necessary. The patient must learn how to insufflate the oesophagus with air, how to retain it there and, more importantly, how to release a small volume of air under control to vibrate the pharyngeal mucosa. Oesophageal speech training is time consuming and, occasionally, the training opportunities may not meet the requirement of the patient. The tedious learning procedure can be frustrating, although determination and perseverance are key factors for success (Table 6.2). Unfortunately, even the highly motivated patient may not be able to acquire the ability effectively. It has been reported that only 30% of patients are able to employ oesophageal speech as their primary communication modality [1,2]. The quality of oesophageal speech also decreases when other methods of pharyngeal reconstruction have been employed, such as a myocutaneous flap or free jejunal graft [3].

Table 6.1 *Mechanism of sound production*

Type of speech	Vibration source	Vibrator
Oesophageal speech	Air in oesophagus	Pharyngeal mucosa
Voice prosthesis	Pulmonary air	Pharyngeal mucosa
Electrolarynx	Battery-driven motor	'Plastic' diaphragm
Pneumatic device	Pulmonary air	Rubber band within the barrel of the device

Table 6.2 *Oesophageal speech*

Advantages	Disadvantages
No external device required	Long periods of training
Natural speech	Determination to learn
Both hands free	Low-amplitude speech

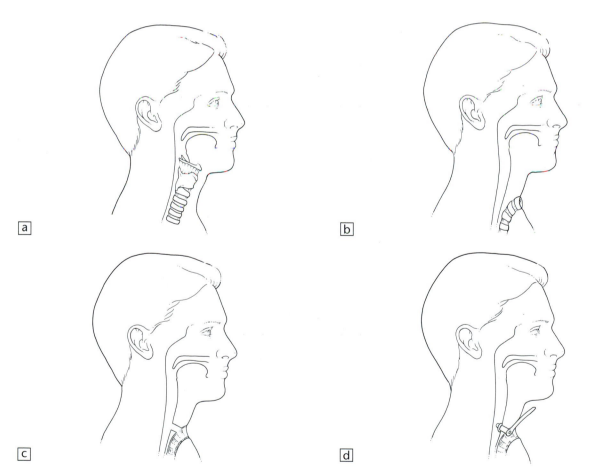

Figure 6.2 Schematic drawing of: (a) normal laryngopharyngeal anatomy; (b) the pharyngeal region following total laryngectomy, showing separation of the trachea from the pharynx; (c) creation of a fistula between pharynx and trachea; and (d) a voice prosthesis placed within the fistula.

Nevertheless, once acquired, oesophageal speech is an effective method of communication. No external device is used as an aid and no maintenance is required. It is not necessary to insert an implant which might induce various tissue reactions and for which care must be exercised for optimal functioning. Both hands are free while using oesophageal speech, there being no need to hold an appliance or to occlude the tracheostomy.

Tracheo-oesophageal puncture

Because the volume of air employed for oesophageal speech is only about one-tenth of the vital capacity of the lung, it is preferable to try and utilize pulmonary air to vibrate the pharyngeal mucosa to produce sound. This can be achieved with the surgical creation of a tract between the trachea and pharynx [4] (Fig. 6.2). On phonation, the tracheostomy is occluded by the thumb, and expiratory air from the lung is diverted through the tract to the pharynx to vibrate the pharyngeal mucosa. An ideal tract should open readily on phonation and close tightly during the passage of saliva or food in order to avoid aspiration. A fistula between the posterior tracheal wall and the pharynx may be created surgically,

at the time of laryngectomy, to facilitate voice restoration (Fig. 6.3).

A surgically constructed fistula tract may have problems. Adequate vibration of the pharyngeal mucosa to produce vowel voice requires an air flow through the tract of at least 50–100 ml/s [5]. If a patent tract permits the flow of this volume of air, its lumen is wide enough for saliva or fluid to run from the pharynx to the trachea and to cause aspiration. Epithelial lining tracts are prone to fibrosis with the development of stenosis following irritation, especially in patients who have received radiotherapy. To circumvent this difficulty, a hollow stent, which has a unidirectional valve within its lumen, can be inserted through the fistula, and this is termed the 'voice prosthesis'. Thus, air can traverse the prosthesis from the lung to the pharynx to vibrate pharyngeal mucosa, and the one-way valve prevents aspiration of fluid. This method of voice restoration was initially carried out after laryngectomy as a secondary procedure, if alternative methods of voice restoration were unsatisfactory [6]. A rigid bronchoscope was inserted into the pharynx with the bevel facing anteriorly, and the slanting lumen of the scope positioned behind the upper part of the posterior tracheal wall. A puncture is made out through the posterior part of the tracheal wall into the pharyngeal lumen (Fig. 6.4). This tract is then dilated gradually to allow the insertion of a size 16 Fr catheter. After a week, when the tract has matured, the voice prosthesis can be inserted. Optimal function of the voice prosthesis under these circumstances depends on the tightness of closure of the inferior constrictor muscle at the time of the primary surgery. The potential for success in using the

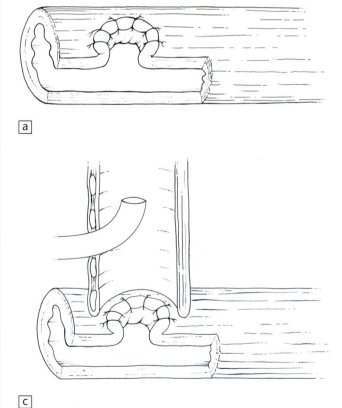

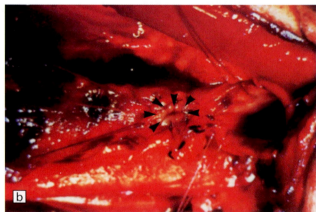

Figure 6.3 Tracheo-oesophageal fistula (Stafieri technique). (a) Schematic drawing of everted oesophageal mucosa. (b) Operative photograph: the oesophageal mucosa is everted through a hole on the anterior wall of the oesophagus and sutured (arrowheads). (c) Schematic drawing showing the segment of oesophagus with the fistula opening sutured to the divided lumen of the trachea.

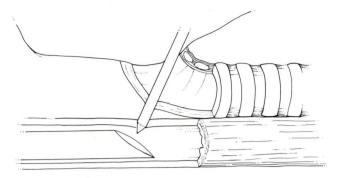

Figure 6.4 Schematic drawing of puncture through the posterior wall of the trachea to create the tracheo-oesophageal fistula.

resection, the creation of a tracheo-oesophageal fistula is frequently carried out at the time of laryngectomy as a primary procedure. On completion of total laryngectomy, a myotomy is made in the cricopharyngeal muscle and extended upwards for half the vertical length of the inferior constrictor (Fig. 6.5). To facilitate the procedure, the muscular coat of the pharynx and the upper oesophagus is stretched or distended. This can be achieved by placing stay sutures at the edge of the pharyngeal wall and the insertion of a finger into the pharyngo-oesophageal lumen to distend the muscular coat. With a scalpel or scissors, only the muscular coat is divided, the mucosal layer being left intact. The myotomy is usually carried over the posterior wall of the pharynx and the upper oesophagus; its lower limit should be below the pharyngeal end of the tracheo-oesophageal fistula.

voice can be predicted by the oesophageal insufflation test, performed before tracheo-oesophageal puncture [7].

With improved experience, and the reluctance of the patient to undergo a secondary procedure after the initial

Voice prostheses

The two commonly used voice prostheses are the Blom Singer and the Provox voice prosthesis.

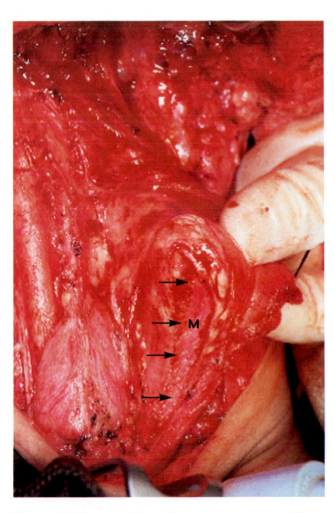

Figure 6.5 Myotomy of the cricopharyngeal muscles. The muscle is divided (arrows) showing the mucosa (M).

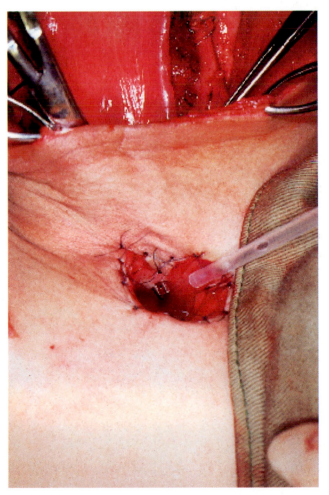

Figure 6.6 The tip of forceps is inserted through the oesophageal and post-tracheal walls.

Blom Singer voice prosthesis

To create a fistula for this prosthesis, after the myotomy, a curved forceps is inserted into the lumen of the pharynx and pushed anteriorly to elevate a small portion of the posterior tracheal wall. A small wound is made on the posterior tracheal wall over the tip of the forceps (Fig. 6.6). The forceps are then used to grasp the tip of a catheter and withdraw it into the pharyngeal lumen (Fig. 6.7). This catheter is then guided down the oesophagus and can be used as a feeding tube during the postoperative period. When the tract has epithelialized, usually by the tenth postoperative day, then the Blom Singer voice prosthesis of an appropriate length can be inserted on removing the catheter.

The diameter of the Blom Singer voice prosthesis ranges from 14 to 20 Fr in size, and the one-way valve, in early versions, was in the form of a 'duckbill'. In view of the size of the prosthesis, together with the particular valve design, more pressure is required to direct the pulmonary air to vibrate the pharyngeal mucosa. The next generation model has a modified unidirectional valve with a low-pressure system so that minimal pressure is required for air to flow from the trachea to the pharynx for sound production (Fig. 6.8). There is much wider acceptance of this type of voice prosthesis. However, to maintain function of the Blom Singer voice prosthesis, it must be removed for cleaning daily, or at least two to three times each week.

Provox voice prosthesis

When this voice prosthesis is inserted at the primary operation, the procedure is slightly more complicated. After the myotomy, a hollow metal tube is inserted into the pharyngeal lumen and its bevel is turned towards the posterior tracheal wall. A curved trochar and cannula is inserted through the upper part of the posterior tracheal wall into hollow of the metal tube and, effectively, the

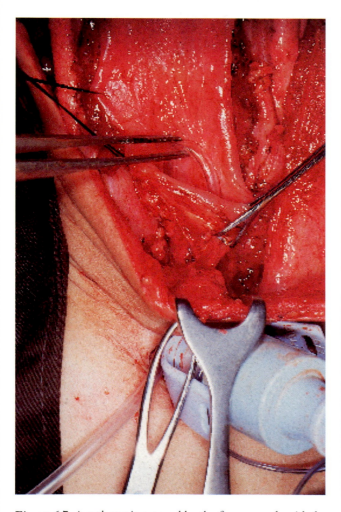

Figure 6.7 A catheter is grasped by the forceps and guided into the oesophagus for feeding during the postoperative period. This catheter also serves to splint the fistula tract.

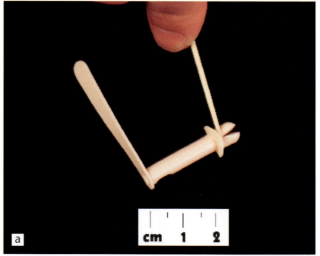

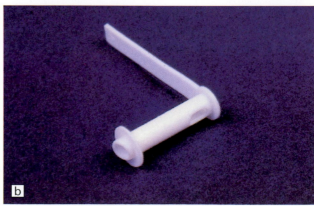

Figure 6.8 Blom Singer voice prosthesis. (a) Duckbill type. (b) Low-pressure design with a unidirectional valve.

pharyngeal lumen (Fig. 6.9). A catheter with a catch is inserted through the lumen of the cannula into the opened pharynx and into the surgical wound. The Provox voice prosthesis is attached to the hole at the end of the catheter (Fig. 6.10). On withdrawing the catheter, the voice prosthesis is delivered through the posterior tracheal wall to be placed in an optimal position (Fig. 6.11).

The lumen of the Provox voice prosthesis is 8 mm in diameter, and this is much wider than the Blom Singer design. In view of its large sized lumen and the design of the flap-like unidirectional valve, very little pressure is required for the Provox to function. The Provox voice prosthesis is designed to be indwelling, i.e. once it is inserted, it does not require frequent removal for cleaning. A specially designed brush is employed for cleaning purposes, and the patient simply inserts this through the voice prosthesis from the tracheal end.

The choice of voice prosthesis (see Box 6.1)

When the catheter for splinting the tract is removed, the appropriate-sized Blom Singer voice prosthesis should be inserted immediately. If the fistula tract is left alone, it rapidly decreases in size and may close within 1–2 days. Adequate attention from the medical staff for care of the fistula and the voice prosthesis is required, especially in the early stages. During the early postoperative period, the patient must become familiar with the care of the prosthesis. He or she must be advised that if the prosthesis slips out and there is difficulty in reinsertion, a catheter should be used to splint the fistula, and medical consultation sought. The patient should be educated as to the careful insertion and changing of the prosthesis at home. Adequate visual ability and hand coordination is required to carry out the procedure.

The Provox voice prosthesis does not have this problem as once placed in position, it is seldom dislodged and does not require frequent changing. Cleaning of the prosthesis is also simple and can be carried out by the patient with ease. When a change of the Provox prosthesis is required however, it is more complicated than for the Blom Singer prosthesis, and medical staff assistance is mandatory.

Box 6.1 *Points to consider in choosing a voice prosthesis*

- The age of the patient
- The patient's ability to care for the prosthesis
- Medical manpower involved in changing the prosthesis
- Surgical expertise available
- The cost of the prosthesis
- The frequency of replacing the prosthesis

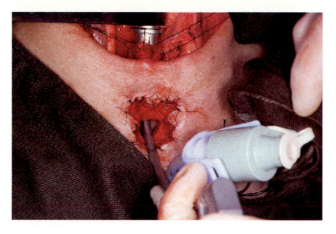

Figure 6.9 The trochar and cannula are inserted through the post-tracheal wall into the lumen of the hollow metal tube which is placed within the pharyngeal lumen.

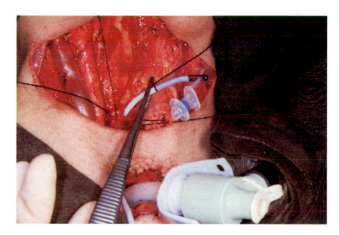

Figure 6.10 A Provox prosthesis attached to the catheter which is inserted through the tract is guided into position on being withdrawn.

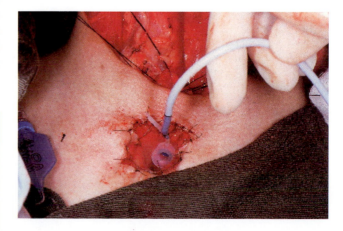

Figure 6.11 A Provox voice prosthesis placed in the fistula with one flange lying in the post-tracheal wall, near the upper end of the terminal tracheostome.

The life span of the Blom Singer voice prosthesis may be up to 6 months, while the Provox may last for a year. A common reason for the need for a new prosthesis is leakage of fluid during swallowing. The unidirectional valve within the prosthesis may not function correctly, either because of wear and tear or from damage due to colonization by fungi.

In addition to the cost and the time required in caring for the prosthesis, management of the fistula tract when the prosthesis is no longer required should also be taken into consideration. After removal of a Blom Singer prosthesis the fistula tract usually closes within a few days. When fistula opening is persistent, only a minor procedure is required for its closure. However, following the removal of a Provox prosthesis the fistula tract is more problematic and a formal surgical procedure is usually required for its closure.

The Blom Singer voice prosthesis is currently used for relatively young patients who are able to care for the tract and change the prosthesis. Once oesophageal speech is learned, the prosthesis can be removed and the sequelae are minimal. The Provox voice prosthesis is recommended for older patients who can make use of this soon after operation. The demand on the patient to care for the Provox prosthesis is minimal, and it needs to be changed by medical staff only once a year.

Complications of voice prostheses

Placement of the voice prosthesis frequently causes infection and irritation at the tracheostomy site. These contribute to the increased incidence of stomal stenosis in patients with voice prosthesis insertion [8]. The tracheostomy may be narrowed to such an extent that, with the prosthesis in place, airway patency may be affected. In these circumstances, revision of the tracheostomy is frequently necessary. The Blom Singer prosthesis is sometimes dislodged and the patient may aspirate the voice prosthesis into the tracheobronchial

tree. However, when this situation is recognized, retrieval of the prosthesis with a bronchoscope is not difficult.

A more serious problem is leakage of saliva or fluid around the voice prosthesis, leading to aspiration. This happens more frequently in patients who have undergone radiation treatment of the primary malignancy. The tissues may not heal as desired, resulting in the formation of a fistula tract that is wider than the prosthesis. The prosthesis must be removed and a catheter used to splint the tract. Tissue around the tract usually contracts after a few days, after which the prosthesis may be reinserted. On the rare occasion that the tract does not close, then a surgical procedure should be carried out to facilitate its healing and narrowing (Table 6.3).

Efficacy of voice prostheses

Despite problems associated with voice prostheses, these are still used frequently as the procedure of choice for voice rehabilitation after total laryngectomy. This is largely because of the advantages of tracheo-oesophageal speech over other methods of voice rehabilitation. The advantages include simple and short training periods, the ability to produce louder sounds with a longer phonatory period, and that the speech produced is more intelligible [2,9]. Patients using tracheo-oesophageal speech can produce higher-intensity sounds and more words per minute than is possible with other methods of voice rehabilitation [10]. With the production of louder and a wide dynamic range of sound, patients using a voice prosthesis can even produce tonal languages, as shown in a prospective study [11] (Table 6.4).

Evaluation of the long-term success with the voice prosthesis as a primary voice rehabilitation method has ranged from 52% to 90% [12–14]. Some patients may go on to acquire other methods of voice rehabilitation, whereas others may have lost the tract after dislodgement of the prosthesis.

Table 6.3 *Complications of voice prostheses and their management*

Problem	Solution
Leakage of saliva	Use a new prosthesis
Dislodged prosthesis	Retrieval and re-insertion
Stenosis of tracheostome	Revision of tracheostome
Persistent fistula after removal of prosthesis	Surgical closure of fistula

Table 6.4 *Advantages and disadvanatges of voice prostheses*

Advantages	Disadvantages
Loud sound	Surgical procedure involved
Long phonatory period	Care of voice prosthesis required
Intelligible speech	Complications may develop
Moderate cost of prosthesis	New models may be expensive

External voice aid devices

The 'electrolarynx'

The most commonly used external voice aid device is the 'electrolarynx', in which the sound is generated through the vibration of a diaphragm driven by a battery. The electrolarynx is applied to an area over the neck, and the generated sound is transmitted to the pharynx, after which it is further modified by the intact articulators, teeth, tongue and lips to become intelligible speech. Sometimes, the neck tissue is thick or fibrotic following surgery and radiotherapy, and transmission of sound to the pharynx is then not effective. A mouthpiece may be attached to the electrolarynx and the generated sound transmitted directly to the mouth where it is modified as speech (Fig. 6.12).

Pneumatic voice aids

The body segment of the pneumatic voice aid contains an adjustable rubber band, and one end of the segment is funnel-shaped. The other end of the device is connected to a mouthpiece. The funnel end of the pneumatic device is placed over the tracheostomy, and expiratory air vibrates the rubber band in the body segment to generate sound.

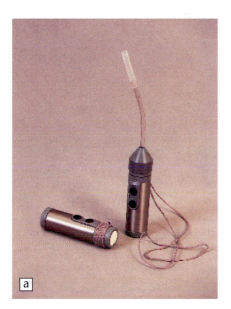
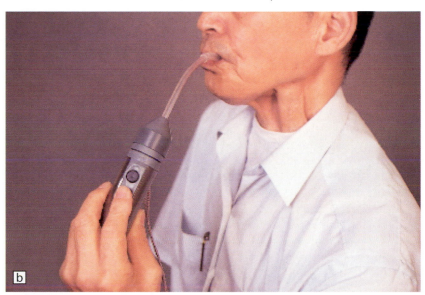

Figure 6.12 (a) Electrolarynx. (b) Electrolarynx with a mouthpiece in use.

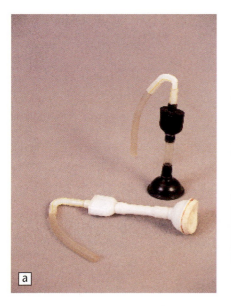
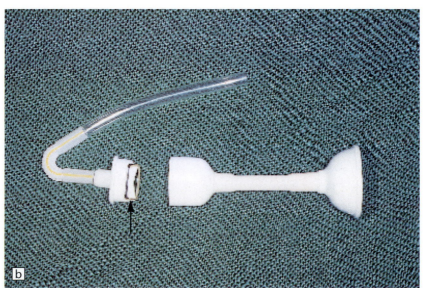

Figure 6.13 (a) Two pneumatic voice aids. (b) Pneumatic voice aid disconnected; the vibrator is within the barrel (arrow).

The sound is then transmitted through the mouthpiece to the mouth and is converted to speech by the articulators. The length of the rubber band can be varied to produce different pitches, and gender-based sound characteristics can be imitated to some extent (Fig. 6.13).

Speech generation with external voice aids

Minimal training with external voice aid devices is required to produce intelligible speech. When available, the device contributes to the production of speech for someone who has completely lost the ability to communicate with others by normal vocalization.

One drawback with the speech of a patient using the electrolarynx is that it is monotonous and sounds 'mechanical'. The quality of the speech, although intelligible, does not sound natural and this limits the device's acceptability. As the device is driven by battery, power failure or structural malfunctioning makes it somewhat unreliable. In addition, as the device has to be applied to suitable areas on the neck, the neck tissues must be pliable and soft in order for it to function adequately. The use of the mouthpiece adversely affects the external image of the patient as it does not appear normal when talking in a crowd; the same is true for the pneumatic device.

Although speech produced with the pneumatic device is more natural, the use of the mouthpiece frequently leads to problems of hygiene, in addition to its awkward appearance. These external devices cannot be used when both hands are occupied. The purchase of the device and its maintenance also have financial implications, especially in developing countries. It is due to these limitations that external voice aid devices have not gained overwhelming popularity, and they are generally used as a means of

Table 6.5 *Properties of external voice aid devices*

Advantages	Disadvantages
Minimal training required	Cost and maintenance of device
Easy to use	Produces unnatural and mechanical sound
	Have to hold device with hand
	Hygiene problems with pneumatic device
	Appearance of using these devices not appealing

vocal communication only when other methods of voice rehabilitation have failed (Table 6.5).

Summary

Oesophageal speech is the most natural way to vocalize after total laryngectomy, though long periods of training are required to achieve this. The main disadvantages of oesophageal speech are the low intensity of sound and the short length of sentences.

Voice prosthesis speech rehabilitation does not have these limitations, although a surgical procedure is involved and the patient has to care for the prosthesis. External devices may be used to produce reasonable speech when other methods of voice rehabilitation are not applicable.

References

1. Snidecor JC. Some scientific foundations for voice restoration. *Laryngoscope* 1975; 85: 640–648.

2. Gates GA, Ryan WJ, Cooper JC. Current status of laryngectomy rehabilitation: results of therapy. *Am J Otolaryngol* 1982; 3: 1–4.

3. Gates GA, Hearne EM. Predicting esophageal speech. *Ann Otol Rhinol Laryngol* 1982; 91: 454–457.

4. Amatsu M. A one stage surgical technique for postlaryngectomy voice rehabilitation. *Laryngoscope* 1980; 90: 1378–1386.

5. Smitheran JR, Hixon TJA. A clinical method for estimating laryngeal airway resistance during vowel production. *J Speech Hear Disord* 1981; 46: 138–146.

6. Singer MI, Blom ED. An endoscopic technique for restoration of voice after laryngectomy. *Ann Otol Rhinol Laryngol* 1980; 89: 529–533.

7. Blom ED, Singer MI, Hanmaker RC. An improved esophageal insufflation test. *Arch Otolaryngol Head Neck Surg* 1985; 111: 211–112.

8. Ho CM, Wei WI, Lau WF, Lam KH. Tracheostomal stenosis after immediate tracheoesophageal puncture. *Arch Otolaryngol Head Neck Surg* 1991; 117: 662–665.

9. Blom ED, Singer MD, Hamker RC. A prospective study of tracheoesophageal speech. *Arch Otolaryngol Head Neck Surg* 1986; 112: 440–447.

10. Robbins J, Fisher HB, Blom ED. Selected acoustic features of tracheoesophageal, esophageal, and laryngeal speech. *Arch Otolaryngol Head Neck Surg* 1984; 110: 670–672.

11. Wong SHW, Cheung CCH, Yuen PW *et al*. Assessment of tracheoesophageal speech in a tonal language. *Arch Otolaryngol Head Neck Surg* 1997; 123: 88–92.

12. Wong SHW, Yuen PW, Cheung CCH *et al*. Long-term results of voice rehabilitation after total laryngectomy using primary tracheoesophageal puncture in Chinese patients. *Am J Otolaryngol* 1997; 18: 94–98.

13. Kao WW, Mohr RM, Kimmel CA *et al*. The outcome and techniques of primary and secondary tracheoesophageal puncture. *Arch Otolaryngol Head Neck Surg* 1994; 120: 301–307.

14. Van Weissenbruch R, Albers FWJ. Vocal rehabilitation after total laryngectomy using the Provox voice prosthesis. *Clin Otolaryngol* 1993; 18: 359–364.

CHAPTER seven

Management of
cervical lymph node

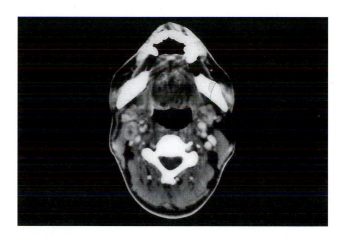

Introduction

The management of cervical lymph nodes and their metastases is important in treatment of carcinoma of the larynx, as the presence of cervical lymph nodes is a significant prognostic factor [1] (Table 7.1). The incidence of metastasis is associated with the size and location of the primary tumour in the larynx. Stage for stage, patients with glottic tumour less often develop cervical lymph node metastases than do those patients with cancer of the supraglottis [2]. The rationale for treatment of cervical lymph nodes in carcinoma of the larynx is controversial, especially when the nodes are not clinically palpable. In addition, the need for imaging studies to identify subclinical cervical lymph nodes may also vary with the location of the primary tumour.

Treatment options for cervical lymph nodes include either surgery or radiotherapy, or both. The selection of a particular treatment mode for a particular patient may need to be individualized, and the choice will depend on various factors, including the patient's wishes, the expertise available at the institute, and which treatment modality is to be employed for the primary tumour (Box 7.1). When surgical treatment is decided upon, the type of neck dissection that is most appropriate for the patient under the circumstances should be selected, and the decision also made whether or not the contralateral neck is to be included in the treatment.

Box 7.1 *Factors that determine the treatment for cervical nodal metastasis in carcinoma of the larynx*

- Patient's consent for the treatment options
- Surgical expertise available
- Extent of the primary tumour
- Location of the cervical lymph node
- Treatment given for the primary tumour

The N0 neck

The commonly used definition of N0 neck is the absence of palpable cervical lymph nodes clinically. While earlier studies showed the identification of metastasis by clinical palpation to be only 65–70% accurate [3–5], today – with the advent of techniques such as computed tomography (CT) and magnetic resonance imaging (MRI) – metastasis to neck nodes may be determined with much greater accuracy. Ultrasound examination of the neck, together with ultrasound-guided fine needle aspiration, has also been shown to improve detection of occult neck lymph node metastases [6]. The use of these imaging studies, together with physical examinations, has reduced the incidence of occult metastasis to less than 10% [5–7]. Features of the cervical lymph nodes which show that malignancy might be present include the presence of

Table 7.1 *Outline management of lymph node in patients with carcinoma of the larynx*

N0 neck		
Status of primary tumour	If surgery is employed for primary tumour, treatment for the neck	If radiotherapy is employed for the primary tumour, treatment for the neck
T1, T2 all sites, T3 glottic	Neck not treated	Neck not irradiated (except supraglottic T2)
T3 supra, subglottic, T4 all sites	Selective neck dissection, levels II, III and IV	Neck included in the radiation field
• When the primary tumour crosses the midline, bilateral neck treatment is necessary		
N+ neck		
Surgery is usually employed as, at this N stage, the primary tumour is commonly T3 or above		
Status of lymph node	Type of neck dissection	
N1	Modified neck dissection, the structures close to the lymph node are removed	
N2, N3	Radical neck dissection	
• When the primary tumour crosses the midline, bilateral neck treatment is necessary		

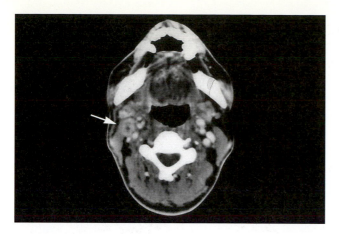

Figure 7.1 Computed tomography of the N0 neck showing a lymph node with central necrosis (arrow). This suggests the presence of malignant cells in the node.

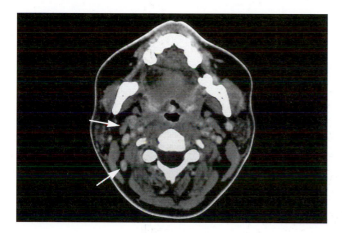

Figure 7.2 Computed tomography of the N0 neck, showing enlarged lymph nodes in the neck (arrows). This suggests the presence of malignant cells in some of the nodes.

central necrosis in the nodes (Fig. 7.1), evidence of involvement of tissue around the node, an enlarged lymph node of more than 1.5 cm diameter, and also when a group of surrounding lymph nodes are affected (Fig. 7.2). Computed tomography or MRI of the neck should be performed when it is necessary to document the extent of involvement of the primary tumour, and especially in those patients in whom there is a high likelihood of metastasis occurring to the cervical lymph nodes.

The incidence of occult cervical lymph node metastasis for cancer of the larynx ranges from 20% to 40% [8,9]. The tendency to metastasize varies with the location of the primary tumour, and supraglottic and subglottic tumours more often metastasize to the cervical lymph nodes than does glottic cancer. There is no evidence to support prophylactic treatment of the neck nodes for all patients suffering from carcinoma of the larynx with N0 neck. In general, to avoid overtreating patients, it may be

Box 7.2 *Indications for treatment of N0 neck*

- Treatment is more effective when the tumour load in the node is small
- If the node is not treated, it may metastasize or develop extracapsular spread
- The patient usually agrees when the neck is treated at the same time with the primary tumour
- Once treated, the patient's compliance in close monitoring of the nodes is not necessary
- With the primary carcinoma at certain sites, treatment of N0 neck improves disease control in the neck

justified that treatment to the neck nodes be initiated only when the incidence of occult metastasis is 25% or more [6]. The ultimate goal of treating neck nodes is to reduce their regional recurrence and to improve patient survival. Treatment of neck disease is never totally successful, but the tumour recurrence rate is lower when the N0 neck is treated than when necks with positive metastasis are treated [3]. While it is easier to treat nodes when they are small, a policy of watchful waiting may be disadvantageous in that the tumour may meanwhile extend to the extracapsular tissue. The compliance of patients for regular follow-up should also be taken into account before deciding on a treatment policy (Box 7.2).

Glottic carcinoma

Although the incidence of neck node metastasis is low, treatment failure in the neck is not uncommon when surgery alone is applied to primary carcinoma. Among 59 patients suffering from T3N0 carcinoma and treated with total laryngectomy, the incidence of treatment failure in the neck was 20%. In the same report, when the entire group of 128 T3 and T4 patients was assessed, 54% developed node recurrence in the neck at one stage or another [10]. Thus, the neck in these patients should be treated.

Radiation treatment for the N0 neck in patients suffering from glottic carcinoma is adequate to control the neck disease. This was evidenced by the fact that for those patients given radical radiotherapy for their advanced primary tumour (including the neck), isolated recurrence in the cervical lymph node was rarely seen. Neck node recurrence in these patients was invariably associated with failure at the primary site [11]. It has also been shown that in patients given radiotherapy for glottic carcinoma, when the primary tumour recurred in these patients the incidence of recurrences in the neck was 22% [12]. Thus, in glottic carcinoma the recommendation is to remove the nodes from N0 necks when surgical salvage is carried out after radiotherapy.

When surgery is performed in those patients with advanced primary glottic carcinoma, the N0 neck on the side of the lesion should be treated electively. Selective neck dissection to remove the lymph nodes in levels II, III and IV as a staging procedure is indicated (Fig. 7.3). If the primary tumour crosses the midline, then bilateral selective neck dissection should be carried out. The associated morbidity is low, and when histology of the specimen reveals metastatic nodes, then further post-operative radiotherapy may be given depending not only on the number of lymph nodes involved but also on whether extracapsular spread was identified.

Supraglottic carcinoma

It is generally considered that the delivery of 4500–5000 cGy of external radiation to clinically negative necks is adequate to eradicate occult tumour cells in the nodes [12,13]. It is difficult to assess the results of such

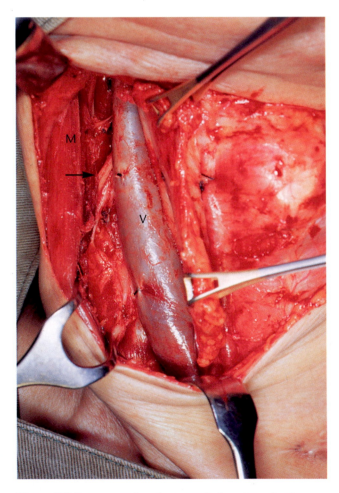

Figure 7.3 Intraoperative photograph showing selective neck dissection of levels II, III and IV on the right side. The sternomastoid muscle (M), internal jugular vein (V) and the spinal accessory nerve (arrow) are preserved, together with lymph nodes in level I and V.

treatment as the incidence of occult positive necks is unknown, and thus many necks that have no metastatic lymph nodes present will be irradiated. The incidence of lymph node recurrence has been used as measurement of success when the primary tumour is controlled with radiation. It is usually acceptable to treat the neck with radiotherapy when radiation is also employed to treat primary supraglottic carcinoma.

In one study where unilateral neck dissection was performed concurrently with surgery for primary supra-glottic tumour, the incidence of failure in the neck at 2 years after surgery was about 20%. Over 90% of these failures occurred in the contralateral neck [14]. When bilateral neck dissection was carried out, the regional failure decreased from 20% to 9%, with no increase in morbidity, although survival improved only marginally [15]. In another study, among 90 patients who had tumour in their neck dissection specimen, 31 subsequently required neck dissection of the contralateral side [16]. Thus, they recommend when surgery is employed as primary treatment for supraglottic carcinoma, selective neck dissection is recommended for the N0 neck on the side of the tumour. The removed lymph nodes should be subjected to frozen section and, if tumour cells are detected, then selective neck dissection should be carried out for the contralateral neck. When surgical salvage is performed in those patients given radiotherapy as primary treatment for supraglottic carcinoma, the same treatment policy for the cervical lymph nodes should be carried out.

Subglottic carcinoma

When all stages are considered, the incidence of metastasis to cervical lymph nodes is estimated to range from 14% to 22% [17,18], though the incidence of metastasis to the paratracheal nodes is 50% or higher [17]. For a subglottic carcinoma, even when no neck dissection has been carried out, the incidence of recurrence in the neck was less than 10% [19]. Neck dissection is usually not performed for subglottic carcinoma with N0 necks, though dissection of lymph nodes around the trachea should be performed (Table 7.2).

The N+ neck

It is generally agreed that when a patient presents with enlarged lymph nodes that are clinically positive, then surgical treatment should be performed. This is because in cases of carcinoma of the larynx that have metastasized to the cervical lymph nodes, the primary tumour is usually T3 or T4. To give these patients radiotherapy – the aim being to preserve the function of speech – is not practical. The optimal treatment for these patients should be

Table 7.2 *Selection of treatment options for N0 neck in carcinoma of larynx*

Location of primary tumour	Radiotherapy	Surgery
Supraglottic	Yes, when primary tumour is treated with radiation. Both sides when tumour crosses the midline	Selective neck dissection removing levels II, III and IV. Both sides when tumour crosses the midline
Glottic	Yes, when primary tumour is treated with radiation (>T3). Both sides when tumour crosses the midline	Selective neck dissection removing levels II, III and IV. Both sides when tumour crosses the midline
Subglottic	Not given	Not performed

surgical resection of the primary tumour and cervical lymph nodes, followed by postoperative radiotherapy.

Types of neck dissection

The Sloan-Kettering Memorial Group has categorized (on an anatomic basis) all lymph nodes in the neck to six regions. Each individual region is named as a level in accordance with its location and its drainage territory of certain anatomical structures [20]:

- Level I. Those lymph nodes within the triangle bounded by the lower border of the mandible, and the digastric muscle. The submandibular gland belongs to this level.
- Level II. The upper jugular group, which includes lymph nodes around the upper region of the internal jugular vein, under the cover of the sternomastoid muscle, extending from the bifurcation of the carotid artery (surgical landmark) or the hyoid bone (clinical landmark) to the base of the skull.
- Level III. The middle jugular group, which includes all lymph nodes under the cover of the middle portion of the sternomastoid extending from the bifurcation of the carotid artery superiorly down to the omohyoid muscle (surgical landmark) or the cricothyroid notch (clinical landmark).
- Level IV. The lower jugular group includes those nodes located around the lower internal jugular vein under the cover of the sternomastoid muscle extending from the omohyoid muscle superiorly to the clavicle inferiorly.
- Level V. The posterior triangle group includes lymph nodes located along the lower part of the spinal accessory nerve between the posterior border of the sternomastoid muscle and the anterior border of the trapezius muscle. The lower boundary is the lateral aspect of the clavicle (Fig. 7.4).

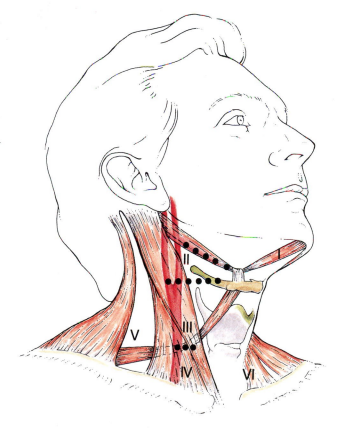

Figure 7.4 Schematic diagram showing the various levels of distribution of lymph nodes in the neck. The operative landmarks, including bifurcation of the carotid artery and inferior belly of the omohyoid muscle, are shown in red. The surface landmarks, including the greater cornu of the hyoid bone and the cricothyroid notch, are shown in green.

- Level VI. Anterior compartment lymph nodes include those that surround the midline visceral structures of the neck extending from the hyoid bone to the suprasternal notch.

Radical neck dissection to remove all lymph nodes in the neck (i.e. all six levels with the sternomastoid muscle, internal jugular vein and the accessory nerve) is the standard oncological treatment to clear the neck of malignant nodes. The operation itself is associated with some mortality and significant morbidity. The incision used for the radical neck dissection should be placed to avoid necrosis of the neck skin flap. Commonly, parallel neck incisions are used and the upper incision extends across the midline to facilitate the laryngectomy (Fig. 7.5). Particular attention should be paid to the thoracic duct when neck dissection is carried out on the left side. Inadvertent injury of the duct and its branches may lead to the formation of chylous fistula and persistent drainage of lymph through the neck wound. The identification and ligation of the thoracic duct at the junction of the left internal jugular vein and the subclavian vein where it joins the venous system will prevent this morbidity (Fig. 7.6). When radical neck dissection is performed with the total laryngectomy, then the carotid artery is exposed. Any leakage from the pharyngeal closure may lead to infection and possible rupture of the carotid artery. On completion of radical neck dissection, the levator scapulae muscle can be lifted and turned medially to cover the entire carotid artery to prevent this serious complication (Fig. 7.7).

The most common adverse outcome of this surgery is the shoulder syndrome. This is an inability to raise the arm, and occurs as a result of the trapezius muscle being paralysed due to removal of the accessory nerve. Movement of the head is also affected following removal of the sternomastoid muscle, and unpleasant swelling and discoloration of the lower face may occur due to compensatory subcutaneous venous dilatation following removal of the internal jugular vein. These functional defects, in association with the cosmetic disfiguration, may limit the patient's ability to work or to engage in sports activities, as well as interfering with their psychological well-being (Box 7.3).

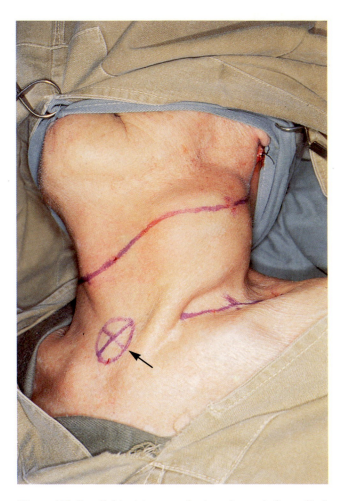

Figure 7.5 Parallel incisions marked on the neck for radical neck dissection together with total laryngectomy. The site of the terminal tracheostomy is also marked (arrow).

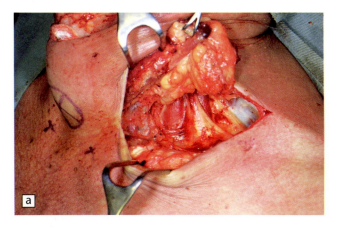

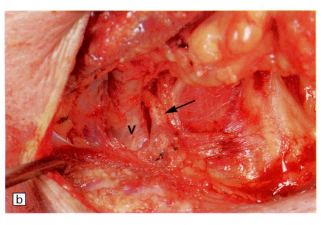

Figure 7.6 (a) Left radical neck dissection exposing the lower medial neck region. (b) Close-up view of the region showing the thoracic duct (arrow) curving laterally to join the venous system at the junction of the left internal jugular vein (V) and the subclavian vein.

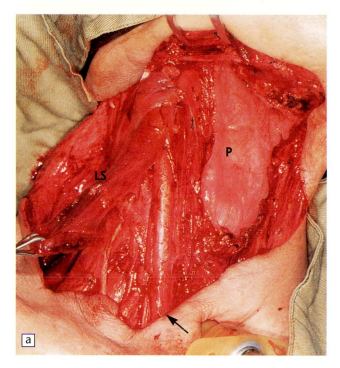

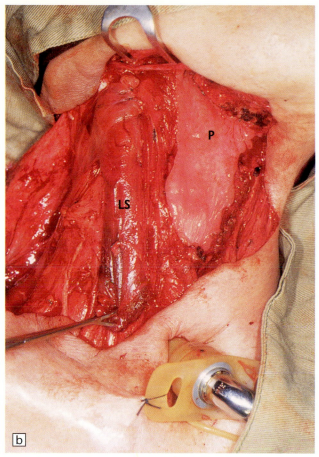

Figure 7.7 (a) The exposed carotid artery (arrow) and the pharyngeal mucosa (P) after radical neck dissection and total laryngectomy. The levator scapulae muscle (LS) is lifted and about to be turned medially to cover the carotid artery. (b) The levator scapulae muscle (LS) is inset to cover the carotid artery. The pharyngeal mucosa (P) is then closed separately.

In view of these complications, a number of modifications of radical neck dissection have been proposed which range from minimal modification – in which only the spinal accessory nerve is spared – to a maximal modification where all nerves, muscles and major vessels are preserved. Many other modifications have been proposed that fall between these two extremes, but the nomenclature is sometimes confusing. Consequently, the Committee for Head and Neck Surgery and Oncology of the American Academy of Otolaryngology, Head and Neck Surgery has proposed a standardization of the types of neck dissection [21] (Table 7.3):

Box 7.3 *Morbidities associated with radical neck dissection*

- Shoulder syndrome, i.e. inability to initiate raising the arm above the head level (the accessory nerve is resected, thus the trapezius muscle is paralysed)
- Reduced movement of the head (sternomastoid muscle removed)
- Lower facial swelling and subcutaneous dilatation of venules (internal jugular vein removed)
- Cosmetic deformity (sternomastoid muscle removed)

- Radical neck dissection. This is the classical radical neck dissection where all the cervical lymph nodes, together with the sternomastoid muscle, internal jugular vein and spinal accessory nerve are removed for tumour clearance.
- Modified radical neck dissection. In this category, all lymph nodes in the neck are removed and one or more of the three major non-lymphatic structures is preserved. Type I dissection refers to the preservation of only the spinal accessory nerve, while type II preserves the nerve with the internal jugular vein. Type III dissection preserves the nerve, vein and also the sternomastoid muscle.
- Selective neck dissection. This involves the removal of lymph nodes in selected levels in the neck, preserving all the major non-lymphatic tissue. The levels selected include the drainage zone for the respective primary tumour. Besides mentioning the levels, the anatomical naming of the selective neck dissections is also used:
  a. Supraomohyoid: includes nodes in levels I, II and III.
  b. Lateral: includes nodes in levels II, III and IV.
  c. Posterolateral: includes nodes in levels II, III, IV and V.
  d. Anterior compartment: includes nodes in level IV.

Table 7.3 *Tissue removed with different types of neck dissection*

Type of tissue removed	Radical neck dissection	Modified neck dissection	Selective neck dissection
Sternomastoid muscle	Yes	Yes, in type I, type II	No
Internal jugular vein	Yes	Yes, in type I	No
Spinal accessory nerve	Yes	No	No
Lymphatic tissue	Yes	Yes	Yes, partly depends on the level of neck dissection

Recommendation

It has been shown that it is rare for metastases from carcinoma of the larynx to go to levels I and V [22,23]. It is thus possible to carry out selective neck dissection for the N+ neck, clearing all nodes of levels II, III and IV, i.e. a lateral selective neck dissection. Modified neck dissections may be carried out in patients where the nodes are close to one of the three structures, the accessory nerve, the internal jugular vein and the sternomastoid muscle. The principle is to remove all the neck disease while not removing unaffected tissue unnecessarily, and to preserve function; all these have been shown to be oncologically sound [24,25].

Radical neck dissection is carried out only when, clinically, the lymph node is fixed – which signifies that it has invaded neck structures. Dissection has also been carried out when the lymph node is larger than 3 cm, or imaging studies have shown an irregular border where extracapsular nodal disease is probably present. It is generally agreed that a conservative form of neck dissection be carried out for N1 disease, and radical neck dissection for N2 and N3 situations [26].

Combined therapy

When the neck dissection specimen reveals the presence of malignant lymph nodes, then whether postoperative radiotherapy should be given is controversial. There was no improvement in survival when radiotherapy was administered for these patients, this is because, the incidence of distant metastasis in retrospective studies were shown to be higher in the postoperative radiotherapy group [27,28]. It was hoped however, that the additional postoperative therapeutic radiation would destroy any microscopic disease left behind inadvertently and those might lead to an increased possibility of tumour recurring in the neck. A high incidence of neck tumour recurrence under this circumstance was devastating to the patient and, though survival was not prolonged, postoperative radio-

therapy had contributed to a better control of lymph node recurrence in the neck [29]. This situation was especially evident when radiotherapy was used to treat the primary tumour bed after laryngectomy. The neck should be included in the postoperative radiation field.

Summary

Correct management of cervical lymph nodes in patients suffering from laryngeal carcinoma is important as these are of prognostic significance. In general, when the primary tumour is treated surgically, then the neck may also be managed surgically. When radiotherapy is employed for the management of the laryngeal cancer, the neck may be included in the radiation field.

For patients with N0 neck, when glottic cancer is small, the neck may be left alone; otherwise for all T3 glottic and all supraglottic laryngeal carcinoma, the cervical lymph nodes must be treated. Surgical treatment should be selective neck dissection of levels II, III and IV on the side of the malignancy, and if this crosses the midline then the contralateral neck should also be dissected. As subglottic carcinomas rarely metastasize to the cervical nodes, the neck may be left alone, though subsequent close monitoring of the patient is essential.

For patients with N+ neck, surgical treatment is usually employed, as the primary tumour is generally of stage T3 or above. For those with N1 neck, a modified neck dissection on the side of the lesion is adequate in order to eradicate the tumour, and radical neck dissection is reserved for N2 and N3 disease. Similarly, when the primary tumour crosses the midline, then the contralateral neck will require treatment.

When surgery is employed as the primary treatment for the tumour in the larynx and neck, postoperative radiotherapy should be instituted when the neck dissection specimen shows the presence of tumour in more than one lymph node or extracapsular spread is present.

References

1. Marks JE, Breaux S, Smith PG *et al*. The need for elective irradiation of occult lymphatic metastases from cancers of the larynx and pyriform sinus. *Head Neck Surg* 1985; 8: 3–8.

2. Till JE, Bruce WR, Elwan A *et al*. A preliminary analysis of the end results for cancer of the larynx. *Laryngoscope* 1975; 85: 259–275.

3. DeSanto LW, Holt JJ, Beahrs OH, O'Fallen WM. Neck dissection: is it worthwhile? *Laryngoscope* 1982; 92: 502–509.

4. van Den Brekel MW, Castelijns JA, Stel HV *et al*. Detection and characterization of metastatic cervical adenopathy by MR imaging: comparison of different MR techniques. *J Comput Assist Tomogr* 1990; 14: 581–589.

5. Friedman M, Mafee MF, Pacella BL *et al*. Rationale for elective neck dissection in 1990. *Laryngoscope* 1990; 100: 54–59.

6. van Den Brekel MW, Stel HV, Castelijns JA *et al*. Lymph node staging in patients with clinically negative neck examinations by ultrasound and ultrasound-guided aspiration cytology. *Am J Surg* 1991; 162: 362–366.

7. Stevens MH, Harnsberger R, Mancuso AA *et al*. Computed tomography of cervical lymph nodes: staging and management of head and neck cancer. *Arch Otolaryngol* 1985; 111: 735 –739.

8. Ali S, Tiwari RM, Snow GB. False positive and false negative nodes. *Head Neck Surg* 1985; 8: 78–82.

9. Farrar WB, Finekelmeier WR, McCabe DP *et al*. Radical neck dissection: is it enough? *Am J Surg* 1988; 156: 173–176.

10. Razack MS, Maipang T, Sako K *et al*. Management of advanced glottic carcinomas. *Am J Surg* 1989; 158: 318–320.

11. Karim AB, Kralendonk JH, Njo KH *et al*. Radiation therapy for advanced (T3-T4 N0-3 M0) laryngeal carcinoma: the need for a change of strategy. A radiotherapeutic viewpoint. *Int J Radiat Oncol Biol Phys* 1987; 13: 1625–1633.

12. Mendenhall WM, Million RR. Elective neck irradiation for squamous cell carcinoma of the head and neck: analysis of time-dose factor and causes of failure. *Int J Radiat Oncol Biol Phys* 1986; 12: 741– 746.

13. Chow JM, Levin BC, Krivit JS, Applebaum EL. Radiotherapy or surgery for subclinical cervical node metastases. *Arch Otolaryngol Head Neck Surg* 1989; 115: 981–984.

14. Lutz CK, Johnson JT, Wagner RL, Myers EN. Supraglottic carcinoma: patterns of recurrence. *Ann Otol Rhinol Laryngol* 1990; 99: 12–17.

15. Weber PC, Johnson JT, Myers EN. The impact of bilateral neck dissection on pattern of recurrence and survival in supraglottic carcinoma. *Arch Otolaryngol Head Neck Surg* 1994; 120: 703–706.

16. DeSanto LW, Magrina C, O'Fallon WM. The second side of the neck in supraglottic cancer. *Otolaryngol Head Neck Surg* 1990; 102: 351–361.

17. Harrison DFN. The pathology and management of subglottic cancer. *Ann Otol Rhinol Laryngol* 1971; 80: 6–12.

18. Stell PM, Tobin KE. The behavior of cancer affecting the subglottic space. *Can J Otolaryngol* 1975; 4: 612–617.

19. Shaha AR, Shah JP. Carcinoma of the subglottic larynx. *Am J Surg* 1982; 144: 456–458.

20. Robbins RT, Medina J E, Wolfe GT *et al*. Standardization neck dissection terminology: official report of the Academy's Committee for Head and Neck Surgery and Oncology. *Arch Otolaryngol Head Neck Surg* 1991; 117: 601–605.

21. Shah JP, Strong E, Spiro RH, Vikram B. Neck dissection: current status and future possibilities. *Clin Bull* 1981; 11: 25–33.

22. Shah JP. Patterns of cervical lymph node metastasis from squamous carcinoma of the upper aerodigestive tract. *Am J Surg* 1990; 160: 405–409.

23. Li XM, Wei WI, Guo XF *et al*. Cervical lymph node metastatic patterns of squamous carcinoma in the upper aerodigestive tract. *J Laryngol Otol* 1996; 110: 937–941.

24. Feldman DE, Applebaum EL. The submandibular triangle in radical neck dissection. *Arch Otolaryngol* 1977; 103: 705–706.

25. Skonlik EM, Yee KF, Friedman M, Golden TA. The posterior triangle in radical neck surgery. *Arch Otolaryngol* 1976; 102: 1–4.

26. Lingeman RE, Helmus C, Stephens R, Ulm J. Neck dissection: radical or conservative. *Ann Otol Rhinol Laryngol* 1977; 86: 737–744.

27. Fletcher GH. Basic principles of the combination of irradiation and surgery. *Int J Radiat Oncol Biol Phys* 1979; 5: 2091–2096.

28. Schuller DE, McGuire WF, Krause CJ *et al*. Adjuvant cancer therapy of head and neck tumors: increased survival with surgery alone versus combined therapy. *Laryngoscope* 1979; 89: 582–594.

29. Jesse RH, Fletcher GH. Treatment of the neck in patients with squamous cell carcinoma of the head and neck. *Cancer* 1977; 39: 868–872.

CANCER OF THE HYPOPHARYNX

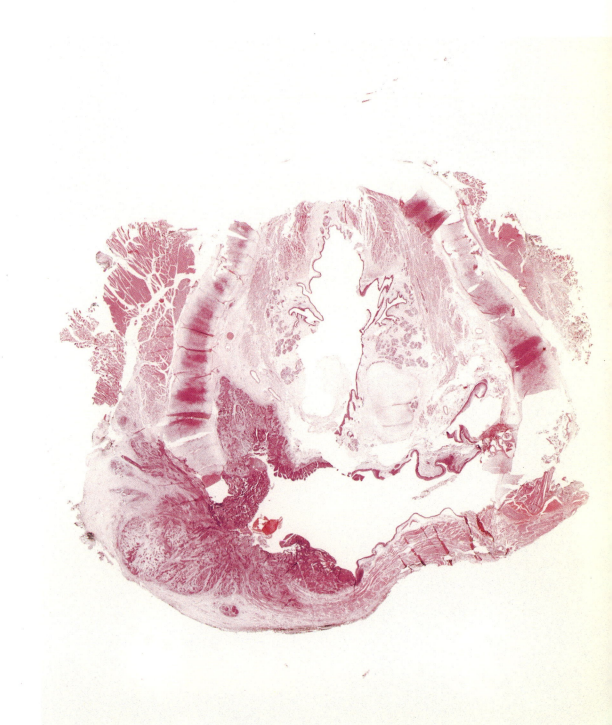

CHAPTER eight

Evaluation of
hypopharyngeal cancer

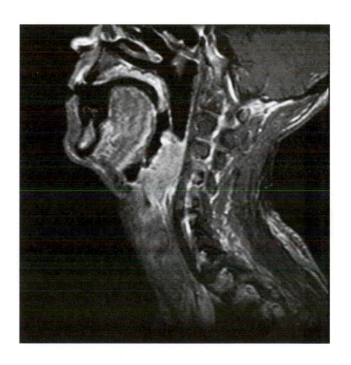

Introduction

The hypopharynx is the name given to the lower portion of the pharynx. Structurally, the hypopharynx is essentially a mucosa-lined muscular tube. The inferior constrictor forms the muscular wall of the hypopharynx and is composed of two portions:

- the thyropharyngeus, which arises from the oblique line of the thyroid cartilage; and
- the cricopharyngeus, which arises from the cricoid cartilage.

The muscle fibres insert in to the median raphe posteriorly to form a complete muscular tube. Mucous membrane lining the pharyngeal wall is composed of stratified squamous epithelium.

Vertically, the hypopharynx extends from the level of the upper border of the epiglottis to the lower border of the cricoid cartilage. It is funnel-shaped, the lumen being wider in its upper part and decreasing as it descends. It is narrowest at its lower end where it joins the cervical oesophagus. Anteriorly, the hypopharynx opens into the sloping laryngeal inlet while, posteriorly, the pharyngeal wall extends from the third to the sixth bodies of the cervical vertebrae (Fig. 8.1).

Anatomically, the hypopharynx is divided arbitrarily into three regions. The piriform fossae are two recesses, one lying on each side of the laryngeal inlet. The medial wall of the fossa is composed of the lower part of the aryepiglottic fold, while it is embraced laterally by the medial aspect of the thyroid cartilage ala in front and continues as the lateral wall of the hypopharynx. The postcricoid region is the whole segment of the pharynx extending from the lower border of the arytenoids to its junction with the cervical oesophagus. The third region is the posterior pharyngeal wall that extends from the lower boundary of the oropharynx to the upper margin of the postcricoid region (Fig. 8.1).

Carcinomas arising at this site are mostly squamous cell carcinomas, and these have a high tendency to extend submucosally and also metastasize to the cervical lymph nodes (Box 8.1). The incidence of lymph node metastasis depends on the location of the primary tumour, being 75% for piriform fossa lesions, 60% for posterior pharyngeal

---

Box 8.1 *Characteristics of hypopharyngeal carcinoma*

- Squamous cell carcinoma
- High tendency for submucosal spread
- High incidence of metastasis to cervical lymph node
- Bilateral cervical lymph node metastasis for centrally located lesion

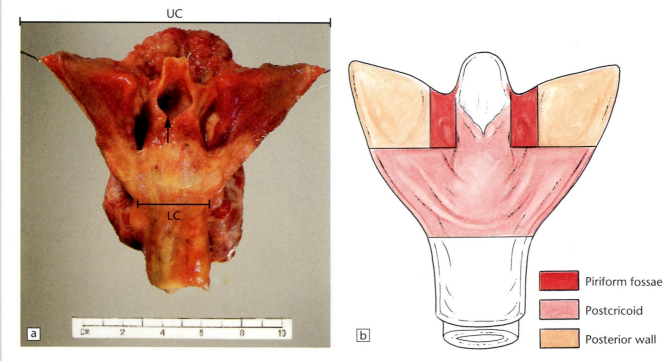

Figure 8.1 (a) Specimen of hypopharynx opened from behind showing a longer circumference at the upper portion (UC) when compared with a shorter circumference (LC) at the lower part. The larynx (arrow) forms the anterior wall of the hypopharynx. (b) Schematic drawing of the hypopharynx, showing the different regions: piriform fossae ( ), postcricoid ( ) and posterior wall ( )).

wall lesions, and 40% when the main tumour bulk is in the postcricoid region. In the latter two locations, regional metastasis tends to be bilateral [1–3].

Besides serving as a conduit for food, the hypopharynx has another important function, i.e. to separate the air and food passages. When food enters the hypopharynx during the third stage of swallowing, the laryngeal inlet is closed while the cricopharyngeal sphincters open appropriately with neuromuscular coordination. Occasionally, after resection of the hypopharynx for tumour clearance, the larynx is also removed, even though the laryngeal function may have been preserved. In this situation, laryngectomy is performed as a prophylactic measure to prevent aspiration.

Clinical assessment

The assessment of a patient suffering from hypopharyngeal carcinoma begins with a check of their general condition. Most patients have some dysphagia that is related to their tumour and are usually nutritionally depleted. Female patients with Plummer–Vinson syndrome may also have anaemia. In addition, many are chronic smokers and alcohol drinkers. Building up patients in preparation for therapy is an essential part of optimal management. In patients with complete dysphagia, rehydration is mandatory, and intravenous feeding may be necessary.

A clinical examination includes palpation of the neck for cervical lymph nodes and assessment of the mobility of the laryngopharynx in relation to the cervical vertebrae. Extension of the carcinoma to the prevertebral muscle, causing fixation, is uncommon but the loss of laryngeal crepitus indicates that there is significant oedema around the hypopharynx, probably associated with a large tumour (Table 8.1).

When tumour extends to involve either the larynx itself or the recurrent laryngeal nerve, hoarseness and chronic aspiration may be evident. Any chest infection must be managed accordingly, and when the tumour leads to obstruction of the air passage, then tracheostomy may be required. The location of the tracheostomy should be planned carefully. It should not be so low that subsequent resection will have to be extended down to the mediastinum, but also it should not be placed too high in order to avoid dissection close to the tumour, as this might lead to recurrence.

Endoscopic assessment

Flexible endoscopy (Table 8.2)
Currently, fibreoptic flexible endoscopes are frequently employed for an initial investigation of the hypopharynx. This is performed under local anaesthesia and any pathology detected is biopsied under direct vision. A flexible end-viewing bronchoscope with a suction channel is the ideal endoscope to use, and this is normally introduced through the nasal cavity to traverse the oropharynx and reach the hypopharynx. Most patients tolerate the procedure better with this approach rather than insertion through the mouth. With adequate application of local anaesthesia, the examination is usually well tolerated, and associated morbidity is minimal.

During the examination, the nasal cavity, the nasopharynx and the oropharynx can be visualized (Fig. 8.2). When the endoscope reaches the hypopharynx, the extent of the lesion can be assessed. Movement of the vocal cords should be noted, together with any direct involvement of the laryngeal apparatus, noting any features that may affect patency of the airway. Whenever there is suspicion of tracheal involvement, then the bronchoscope is introduced through the laryngeal inlet to examine the entire bronchial tree. Biopsies are performed when indicated (Fig. 8.3).

Transverse extension of hypopharyngeal carcinoma can usually be determined by flexible endoscopic examination, whereas confirmation of the vertical extent of the lesion is sometimes difficult. This is particularly challenging

Table 8.1 *Aims of preoperative assessment*

	Evaluation	Management plan
General condition	Nutrition Hydration Anaemia	Preoperative build-up, tube or intravenous feeding
Extent of tumour	Fixation to surrounding tissue Metastasis to cervical lymph node Aspiration status Airway obstruction	Extended resection Neck dissection Chest physiotherapy ± tracheostomy Tracheostomy

Table 8.2 *The 'pros' and 'cons' of flexible and rigid endoscopy*

	Flexible endoscope	Rigid endoscope
Anaesthesia	Local	General
Assessment	Horizontal extent of tumour Mobility of vocal cords	Both horizontal and vertical extent of tumour Postcricoid area
Additional examination	Nasopharynx Tracheobronchial tree Oesophagus	Tracheobronchial tree Oesophagus
Biopsy	Small tissue bulk as limited by the size of biopsy forceps	Large tissue bulk obtained under direct vision
Other applications	Guide the insertion of nasogastric tube	Test mobility of tumour against prevertebral tissue
Risks	Minimal	Low risk of perforating the hypopharynx
Imaging quality	Good	Excellent

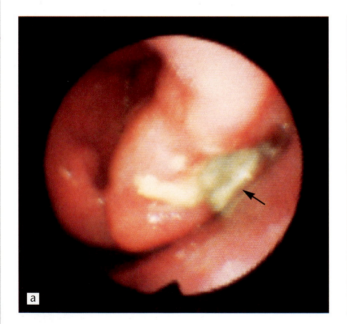
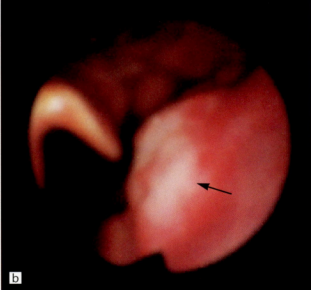

Figure 8.2 Flexible endoscopic examination. (a) Carcinoma at piriform fossa (arrow). (b) Carcinoma arising from the posterior pharyngeal wall (arrow).

when the tumour involves the postcricoid region as the lesion itself obscures endoscopic vision, thus making assessment problematic. It is sometimes helpful to ask the patient to swallow the endoscope into the oesophagus and then, on gradual withdrawal, determine the lower edge of the tumour. This may be facilitated by a flow of air or oxygen at 1–2 litres per minute delivered through the suction channel to distend the oesophagus. In this

way the upper region of the oesophagus can be examined to rule out a synchronous tumour.

The size of the biopsies obtained during flexible endoscopy is limited by the small size of the forceps that can be introduced through the suction channel. Vision through the endoscope may be affected when there is bleeding from the tumour surface as the suction channel may not be large enough to remove all the blood

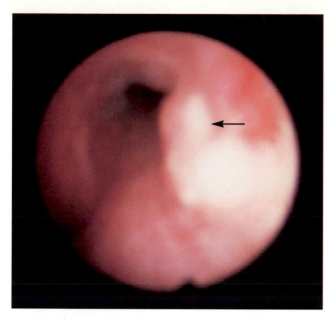

Figure 8.3 Flexible endoscopic examination of the trachea showing a tumour (arrow).

effectively. Despite these limitations, flexible endoscopic examination has additional advantages. In patients with a large tumour leading to obstruction, it may be difficult to introduce a nasogastric tube using conventional methods. These patients usually have significant dysphagia, and enteral feeding is necessary to enable further therapy. Flexible endoscopy enables the manipulation of a guide-wire beyond the tumour under direct vision, and subsequent passage of a nasogastric tube.

Rigid endoscopy

When the vertical extent of the tumour in the hypopharynx cannot be ascertained with flexible endoscopic examination, then rigid endoscopy should be carried out. In this examination, which is performed under general anaesthesia, the tip of a rigid endoscope is introduced behind the postcricoid area. The whole laryngeal apparatus is lifted with the scope to expose the mucosa of the postcricoid region. Close examination of pathology in the region can be performed and adequate biopsy obtained as required (Fig. 8.4).

Rigid endoscopic examination is more traumatic to the patient, and there is also an associated theoretical risk of perforation. Nevertheless, the technique enables a thorough examination of the hypopharynx to be made and, as this is undertaken under general anaesthesia, optimal suction can be utilized to provide a clear field of view for the taking of biopsies.

Imaging studies

The primary aim of imaging studies is to determine the exact three-dimensional extent of tumour involvement so that optimal therapy can be planned.

Lateral plain X-radiographs of the neck in a patient suffering from carcinoma of the hypopharynx may reveal the presence of soft tissue swelling, observed as an increase in the distance between the air column in the trachea and the shadow of the vertebral column (Fig. 8.5). This is only evident in very advanced stage carcinoma when the vertebral body has been eroded or when the

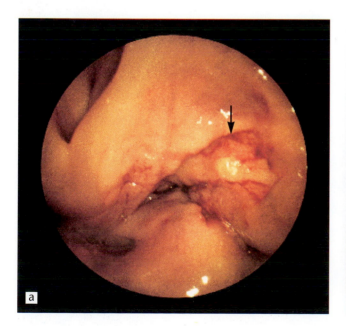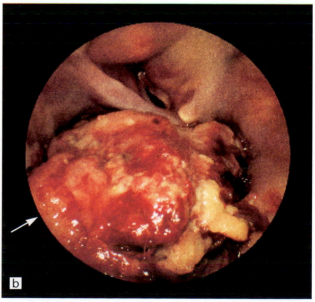

Figure 8.4 Rigid endoscopic examination. (a) Tumour in the postcricoid region (arrow). (b) Large obstructing tumour from the posterior hypopharyngeal wall (arrow).

tumour has ruptured and air is visible in the subcutaneous tissues. Other imaging studies such as contrast laryngography or tomography have more recently been replaced by computed tomography or magnetic resonance imaging.

Contrast studies

In view of the rapid transit of barium through the pharynx, conventional barium swallow may not be very useful for the identification of mucosal pathology. It does, however, give an indication of the patency of the lumen of the pharynx. More useful is an air contrast pharyngogram, which provides detailed delineation of the mucosa of the pharynx. After one or more swallows of a dense suspension of barium, the patient is requested to phonate and then blow through compressed lips. These manoeuvres help to distend the hypopharynx, and any mucosal lesions will be highlighted. One of the limitations of air contrast pharyngography is that although it may show the upper and lateral edges of the tumour well, it rarely outlines the lower border of the lesion (Fig. 8.6).

When there is clinical suspicion of perforation of tumour, water-soluble contrast should be used to demon-strate the fistula. The use of barium may lead to an inflammatory reaction or its retention in the fistula for a long period. Furthermore, when tumour perforation to the tracheobronchial tree is suspected then use of barium or a conventional water-soluble contrast agent may lead to chemical pneumonitis and pulmonary oedema. In these circumstances, a non-ionic and low osmolar water-soluble contrast agent should be employed.

Computed tomography

Computed tomography (CT) is frequently employed to study the extent of hypopharyngeal tumour. It can delineate the extent of submucosal tumour involvement,

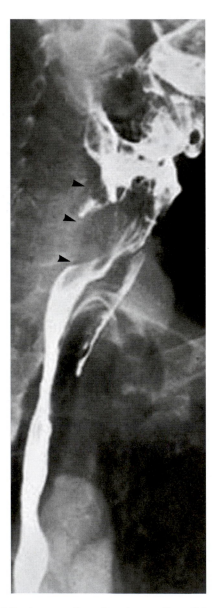

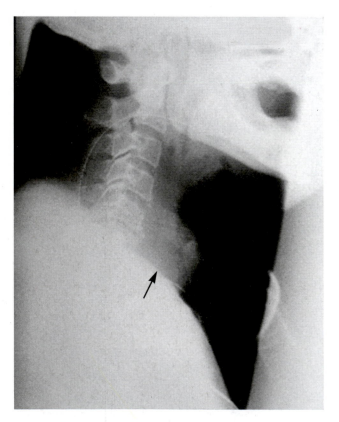

Figure 8.5 Lateral neck X-radiograph showing the increased soft tissue shadow (arrow) in front of the cervical vertebra representing the large tumour in the hypopharynx.

Figure 8.6 Barium swallow showing outline of the tumour (arrowheads) in the hypopharynx.

and also any deep extension to surrounding tissues. The involvement of the larynx and its vicinity by hypopharyngeal tumour can also be visualized [4,5]. For tumours in the piriform fossa, any extension occurring medially that might affect laryngeal structures, and laterally through the thyrohyoid membrane, can be determined and appropriate therapy instituted. For tumours in the posterior pharyngeal wall or the postcricoid area the extent of involvement, particularly whether the lesion crosses the midline, is an important consideration for planning therapy.

Another important use of CT is its ability to detect lymph nodes containing metastatic tumour. Although the density of lymph nodes on CT is similar to that of muscle, malignancy is suspected when nodes are matted together, fascial planes are obliterated, or when a node is larger than 1.5 cm, especially with central necrosis [6,7] (Fig. 8.7). Any suspicious lymph node enlargement may be aspirated with a fine needle for cytological examination. This can be carried out more precisely under CT guidance.

One limitation of CT examination of the primary tumour is that it cannot differentiate between tumour and surrounding tissue oedema. In addition, as pathology can only be examined transversely, its accuracy in the determination of distal end of the tumour is limited. The presence of dental amalgam may also lead to artefacts on CT images.

Magnetic resonance imaging

Magnetic resonance imaging (MRI) shows soft tissue better than CT, and has the additional advantage that

the sagittal plane of examination enables more accurate determination of the vertical extent of tumour in the hypopharynx [9] (Fig. 8.8).

With MRI, the use of intravenous contrast is not necessary to differentiate the vessels from the lymph nodes. On T1-weighted images, lymph nodes are hypodense to fat and isodense or slightly hyperdense to muscle, while on T2-weighted images lymph nodes are isodense when compared with fat and hyperdense to muscle [10]. When there is necrosis within the nodes, these exhibit a reduced signal on T1-weighted images and an increased signal on T2-weighted images. These features provide more clues for identification of tumour in the lymph nodes on MRI (Fig. 8.9).

Limitations of MRI in the imaging of hypopharynx are that it is time-consuming to complete the imaging studies, and a patient's involuntary swallowing may lead to blurred images. In addition, as magnetic fields are used, patients with cardiac pacemakers or clips applied to an intracerebral aneurysm should not be subjected to such an examination.

Summary

A general examination of the patient in relation to his or her stage of the disease is important in order to determine whether nutritional support is necessary. A comprehensive assessment of the extent of hypopharyngeal carcinoma in

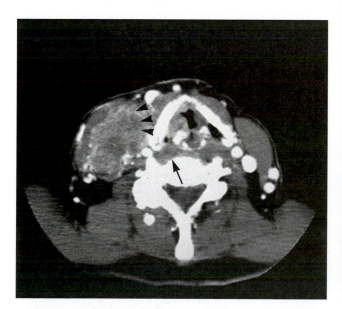

Figure 8.7 Computed tomography scan showing a small tumour in the hypopharynx (arrow) and a large metastatic cervical lymph node (arrowheads).

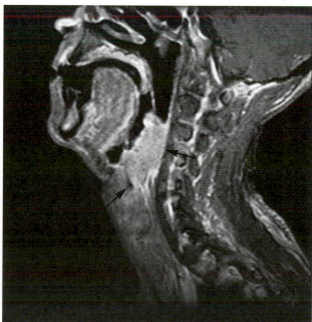

Figure 8.8 Magnetic resonance imaging (MRI) scan showing the extent of tumour in the sagittal plane (arrows). MRI is also used to differentiate the tumour from surrounding soft tissue.

a three-dimensional sense can be achieved with endoscopy and imaging studies.

Endoscopic examination allows direct visualization and biopsy of the tumour, and determination of the extent of tumour on the mucosal surface and its involvement within the aerodigestive tract. Imaging studies further determine the depth of extension of tumour below the mucosal surface, its involvement of surrounding structures, and vertically. CT and MRI are complementary both for the confirmation of the primary tumour and involvement of cervical lymph nodes (Table 8.3).

Accurate staging is required to enable the most appropriate therapy to be administered for the patient suffering from hypopharyngeal carcinoma.

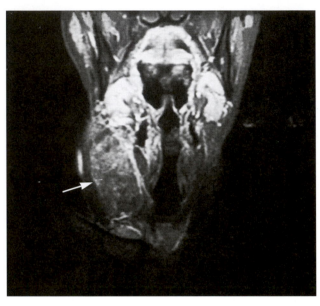

Figure 8.9 Magnetic resonance imaging scan showing metastatic cervical lymph nodes (arrow) in the direct coronal plane.

Table 8.3 *Computed tomography and magnetic resonance imaging in the evaluation of tumour in the hypopharynx*

	Computed tomography	Magnetic resonance imaging
Planes of investigation	Two	Three
Assess bone and cartilage	Good	Poor
Differentiation between tumour and inflammation	Poor	Good
Radiation hazards	Mild	Nil

References

1. Lindberg RD. Distribution of cervical lymph node metastases from squamous cell carcinoma of the upper respiratory and digestive tracts. *Cancer* 1972; 29: 1446–1449.

2. Lefebvre JL, Castelain B, De La Torre JD *et al*. Lymph node invasion in hypopharynx and lateral epilarynx carcinoma: a prognostic factor. *Head Neck Surg* 1987; 10: 14–18.

3. Johnson JT, Bacon GW, Myers EN, Wagner RL. Medial vs lateral wall pyriform sinus carcinoma: implications for management of regional lymphatics. *Head Neck* 1994; 16: 401–405.

4. Mancuso AA, Hanafee WN. A comparative evaluation of computed tomography and laryngography. *Radiology* 1979; 133: 131–138.

5. Asperstrand F, Kolbenstvedt A, Boysen M. Carcinoma of the hypopharynx: CT staging. *J Comput Assist Tomogr* 1990; 14: 72–76.

6. Mancuso AA, Maceri D, Rice D, Hanafee W. CT of cervical lymph node cancer. *Am J Roentgenol* 1981; 136: 381–385.

7. Friedman M, Shelton VK, Mafee M *et al*. Metastatic neck disease. Evaluation by computed tomography. *Arch Otolaryngol* 1984; 110: 443–447.

8. van der Brekel MWM, Valk T, Meyex CT, Snow GB. Cervical lymph node metastasis: assessment of radiological criteria. *Radiology* 1990; 177: 379–384.

9. Lufkin RB, Hanafee WN, Wortham D, Hoover L. Larynx and hypopharynx: MR imaging with surface coils. *Radiology* 1986; 158: 747–754.

10. Jabour BA. Magnetic resonance imaging of metastatic cervical adenopathy. *Top Magn Reson Imag* 1990; 2: 69–75.

CHAPTER nine

Radiotherapy for
hypopharyngeal cancer

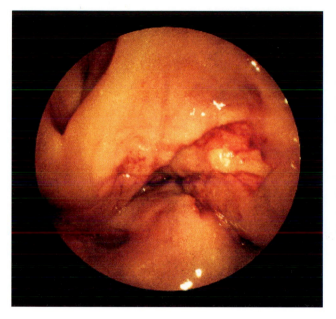

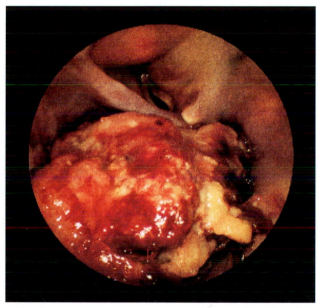

Introduction

In the treatment of hypopharyngeal cancer, the following factors need to be taken into consideration (Box 9.1):

- The propensity for submucosal spread, which may not be detected by endoscopic examination, necessitates treatment of the entire hypopharynx in most cases.
- The site of the tumour; treatment of the adjacent regions of oropharynx and cervical oesophagus may be necessary.
- The propensity for nodal involvement, so that radiotherapy, whether given as primary treatment or given postoperatively, needs also to deal with the cervical lymphatics [1].

Indications for radiotherapy

There is no standard and well-accepted treatment protocol for hypopharyngeal tumours. Treatment depends on the referral pattern and the availability of expertise for surgery and radiotherapy.

For early tumours (T1), radiotherapy and surgery provide similar tumour control, but radiotherapy is associated with better functional (swallowing and speech) and cosmetic results (Table 9.1). For T1 tumours, radiotherapy alone provides local control in 68–80% of cases [2–4]. By comparison, for T2 lesions – even surface lesions – local control after radiotherapy alone was only 57% [5].

For more advanced tumours of the piriform fossa, a combination of surgery and radiotherapy provides an improved cured rate (71%) when compared with radiotherapy (27%) or surgery (53%) alone [6,7]. Although preoperative and postoperative irradiation provide equally good tumour control [8], a postoperative approach is preferred because preoperative radiotherapy is associated with increased complications and morbidities [9].

For tumours of the posterior pharyngeal wall, radiotherapy alone – even with a dose of 70 Gy – is normally associated with poor local control (25%) [10], although much better control (91%) has been reported for T1

tumours [11]. In most cases, a combination of surgery and radiotherapy provides improved local control (49%) when compared with surgery alone (7%). In general, local control of 45–66% has been reported when surgery is followed by postoperative radiotherapy [11].

Postcricoid cancer is associated with a poor result if treated with radiotherapy alone (20%) [12,13], a combination of surgery and postoperative radiotherapy improves local control by 10–20% [14].

For patients with most advanced disease (T4) of the hypopharynx, or those who otherwise are not suitable for surgical treatment because of associated medical illness, radical radiotherapy is usually given.

Radiation techniques

For primary radical radiotherapy, telecobalt units or linear accelerators producing 4–6 MeV photons are ideal to treat the subcutaneous tissues while sparing the overlying skin. Because of the propensity of neck node spread, treatment of posterior and lower neck is usually required (Box 9.2). For treatment of the posterior neck, when the spinal cord tolerance has been reached, electron beams of appropriate energy will be required for treatment. The depth of tissue to be treated may be adjusted

Table 9.1 *Recommended treatment for hypopharyngeal tumours*

Tumor/stage	Treatment
In-situ carcinoma	Surgery or radiotherapy
T1	Surgery or radiotherapy
T2 or T3	Surgery plus postoperative radiotherapy
T4	Radiotherapy (when surgery is considered too extensive)

Box 9.1 *Factors influencing choice of treatment for hypopharyngeal cancers*

- Size and site of the tumour (T stage)
- The availability of expertise in surgery and radiotherapy
- Preference of the patient
- General poor health of the patient may exclude surgery

Box 9.2 *Factors determining radiotherapy field size*

- Size and extent of primary tumour
- Propensity for submucosal spread to oropharynx and cervical oesophagus
- Propensity for nodal involvement
- Need to protect spinal cord from exceeding its radiation tolerance of 45 Gy

by choosing the energy of the electron beam. The thickness of tissue to be treated, and the depth of spinal cord which needs to be protected, are best assessed from a computed tomography (CT) scan.

Treatment is usually given with a pair of lateral opposing fields to cover the primary tumour and the upper two-thirds of the cervical lymphatics. Superiorly, the lateral fields should extend 2–3 cm above the tip of the mastoid to encompass the lymphatics at the base of skull (Box 9.3); inferiorly, the fields should extend 2 cm below the cricoid unless there is further extension inferiorly. Posteriorly, the beam must cover the spinoaccessory chain, and anteriorly the thyroid cartilage, especially when imaging shows the cartilage to have been destroyed by tumour. In the case of more extensive tumour or nodal involvement, a further extension of fields is required to provide a margin of at least 2 cm for the known disease.

After 40–45 Gy treatment, the lateral fields must be reduced in order to protect the spinal cord. The posterior limit of field is reduced to the posterior one-third of the vertebral body, and the posterior neck is treated with electron beams. The total dose to the primary tumour should be 66–70 Gy. If the tumour is not extensive, then the lateral opposing fields may be further reduced after 55–60 Gy at their superior and inferior limits respectively in order to avoid the oropharynx and upper cervical oesophagus. For the posterior neck, treatment is continued with electron beams of the appropriate energy, aiming at a total dose of 55–70 Gy, depending on the extent of the nodal disease.

A matching lower anterior cervical field is used to cover the cervical oesophagus and the lower one-third of the cervical lymphatics (Box 9.4); the apices of the lungs are shielded below the clavicles. A midline shield is required for the lower anterior cervical field after 45 Gy in order to protect the spinal cord.

When a matching lower anterior cervical field is used, a 1-cm shield should be added to the posterio-inferior corner of the lateral opposing cervical fields in order to avoid beam overlap at the spinal cord.

To ensure reproducibility of the treatment position and accuracy of the marks required to direct the beams, and also to avoid putting marks on the patient's skin, a mould is required for all cases. This is usually done under fluoroscopy screening, with patient in the supine position (Box 9.5). A simulator is used to ensure that the alignment of the cervical spine is straight in the anteroposterior and lateral directions. This is to facilitate shielding of the spinal cord from the lateral opposing beams during the second part of treatment. The clinically palpable nodes are marked out on the skin with radio-opaque wire so that they may be localized on the simulator check film. At this point, one option is to have a set of CT scans repeated in the treatment position with the mould; these scans can be used to localize the tumour, as well as for three-dimensional computation of dose distribution. Customized compensators may be required to achieve homogeneity of dose, as the thickness of the target volume often varies considerably between the upper part of the beam and the lower cervical region.

A final verification of accuracy will be performed at the treatment machine, with check films taken to ensure that coverage of the radiation fields is as planned.

Box 9.4 *Additional factors affecting radiotherapy for hypopharyngeal cancers*

- Matching lower anterior cervical field to cover the cervical oesophagus and cervical lymphatics
- Tracheostoma (after surgery or for airway obstruction) is a common site of recurrence
- Propensity of posterior pharyngeal wall tumours to spread to nodes; elective treatment to bilateral cervical lymphatics is required

---

Box 9.5 *Preparations for radiotherapy*

- Patient lying supine, position of head determined under fluoroscopic screening to ensure that the cervical spine is straight
- Cast of head and neck region made in this position
- Option 1 of taking a set of CT scans with this cast for localizing tumour
- Option 2 of taking X-radiograph with simulator for localizing tumour
- Determine the margins required and size of radiation field
- Computation of dose and use of beam compensators if necessary
- Verification by taking check films with treatment machine

Box 9.3 *Landmark structures to be covered with lateral opposing faciocervical field*

- Superior margin 2–3 cm above tip of mastoid to cover lymphatics at skull base
- Inferior margin 2 cm below cricoid
- Posterior margin covers the spinoaccessory chain
- Anterior margin covers the thyroid cartilage
- Further extension of field to give clearance of 2 cm for more extensive tumours

For tumours involving the posterior pharyngeal wall, treatment will be more difficult because of its proximity to the cervical spine; this allows less margin when the lateral fields are reduced after 40–45 Gy. The higher propensity of tumours involving the posterior pharyngeal wall to spread to nodes mandates treatment of bilateral cervical node-bearing areas, and hence the potential risk of overdosing the spinal cord, even with the use of electron beams.

Postoperative irradiation

This is required in most cases except those with earliest tumours, and should be given irrespective of the resection margin or nodal status. Ideally, the patient should be assessed by the surgeon and the radiation oncologist together before surgery (Box 9.6), so that the initial extent of disease is known to the radiation oncologist. At about one week after surgery, when the patient is fit, an assessment should be made by the radiation oncologist and preparation for radiotherapy arranged, the intention being to start treatment at about 3–4 weeks after surgery. Treatment must be postponed when surgical complications such as delayed wound healing are present, but never beyond the sixth week. The assessment includes the surgical operative findings and the pathologist's findings on the surgical specimen, paying particular attention to the sites at risk of failure, such as tumour involvement of the margin or close resection margin.

Treatment will usually consist of large parallel lateral opposing fields to cover the sites of original primary tumour and neck node. Also included are the potential sites of involvement judged from the pattern of spread, as well as the surgical field which is potentially seeded during operation. The surgical scars are marked with metallic wires to localize them on the simulator check film; the purpose of this is to ensure that the scars are covered by radiotherapy. The spinal cord dose should be limited to 45 Gy; when this is reached, the posterior border of the lateral opposing fields will be brought forward to protect the spinal cord. A target dose of 65–68 Gy should be aimed for.

A separate matching lower anterior field is usually required to treat the tracheostomy, which is a common site of relapse, as well as to provide elective irradiation to the lower cervical lymphatics. A midline shield should be added to the lower anterior cervical field after the spinal cord tolerance dose is reached. A target dose of 65–68 Gy should be aimed for.

Treatment in the posterior neck is to be continued with electron beams of appropriate energy, aiming at total dose of 60–68 Gy, depending on the size of original nodal disease. The depth of tissue to be treated may be adjusted by choosing the energy of the electron beam. The thickness of tissue to be treated, and the depth of spinal cord which needs to be protected, are best assessed from a CT scan.

The change in contour and difference in tissue thickness in this part of the body is exaggerated by surgical removal of tissue; thus, the use of tissue compensators to maintain dose homogeneity will be required.

Follow-up after radiotherapy

Following radiotherapy, patients should be seen every 4–6 weeks during the first year, every 2 months in the second year, every 3 months in the third year, and every 4–6 months (or even longer intervals) in the subsequent years (Box 9.7).

As the majority of patients present with advanced disease, most would have been treated using a combination of surgery and radiotherapy. An adequate examination of the pharynx usually requires a fibrescopic examination. Neck examination may be hampered by the fibrosis that results from the combination of neck dissection and radiotherapy.

Unless recurrence at the tumour bed or neck is detected at a very early stage, the chance of successful salvage treatment is small.

Box 9.6 *Postoperative radiotherapy*

- Assessment of patient by surgeon and radiation oncologist before surgery so that extent of tumour known to both teams
- Cast making in preparation of radiotherapy about one week after surgery
- Planning of radiotherapy, taking into consideration operative findings and pathology study of surgical specimen to identify sites at risk of failure
- Start treatment 3–4 weeks after surgery

Box 9.7 *Follow-up after radiotherapy*

- Every 4–6 weeks in the first year, every 2 months in the second year, every 3 months in the third year, every 4–6 months (or longer) in subsequent years
- Adequate examination of pharynx usually requires fibrescope. Examination of neck hampered by fibrosis resulting from combination of surgery and radiotherapy
- Unless recurrence detected very early, chance of successful salvage is small

Complications of radiotherapy

Significant acute mucositis in the pharynx included in the target volume will affect more than 95% of patients, and result in pain that affects swallowing and feeding (Table 9.2). Mucositis manifests as mucosal erythema or whitish patches. Symptoms usually start after 3–4 weeks of treatment and will improve within 2 weeks of completing radiotherapy. Treatment of mucositis is symptomatic with gargles and analgesics, but continued optimal feeding should be encouraged as impairment in nutrition may exacerbate the condition.

An acute skin reaction in the form of erythema and slight pain will occur in many patients, but treatment is again symptomatic.

Fibrosis of the subcutaneous tissue is a common late reaction that occurs 1–2 years after treatment. The severity of the fibrosis is exaggerated by the combination of surgery and postoperative irradiation.

Severe laryngeal oedema and osteochondronecrosis may also occur, especially in patients with advanced tumour who are given high-dose irradiation. However, this is unusual in patients with advanced tumour who are normally treated with combined surgery and radiotherapy.

Hypothyroidism due to irradiation of the thyroid gland occurs in a small percentage of patients; monitoring of thyroxine (T4) and thyroid stimulating hormone (TSH) levels is required to detect subclinical cases of hypothyroidism during follow-up.

Table 9.2 *Acute and late side effects of radiotherapy*

Acute	Late
Mucositis resulting in pain, exacerbated by swallowing. Treatment is symptomatic; the condition will improve spontaneously 2–3 weeks after completion of radiotherapy	Fibrosis of subcutaneous tissue and hypothyroidism. Both will be symptomatic in a small proportion of patients, and will be permanent
Skin reaction. Treatment is symptomatic; the condition will improve spontaneously 2–3 weeks after completion of radiotherapy	Severe laryngeal oedema and osteochondronecrosis in case of primary radiotherapy

References

1. Bataini JP, Brugere J, Bernier J *et al*. Results of radiotherapy treatment of carcinoma of the pyriform sinus: experience of the Institut Curie. *Int J Radiat Oncol Biol Phys* 1982; 8: 1277–1286.

2. Wang C, Schulz M, Miller D. Combined radiation therapy and surgery for carcinoma of the supraglottis and pyriform sinus. *Am J Surg* 1972; 124: 551–554.

3. Dubois JB, Guerrier B, Di Ruggiero JM, Pourquier H. Cancer of the pyriform sinus: treatment by radiation therapy alone and with surgery. *Radiology* 1986; 160: 831–836.

4. Mendenhall WM, Parsons JT, Cassisi NJ, Million RR. Squamous cell carcinoma of the pyriform sinus treated with radical radiation therapy. *Radiother Oncol* 1987; 9: 201–208.

5. Mendenhall WM, Parsons JT, Mancuso AA *et al*. Squamous cell carcinoma of the pharyngeal wall treated with irradiation. *Radiother Oncol* 1988; 11: 205–212.

6. Spector JG, Sessions D, Emami B *et al*. Carcinoma of the aryepiglottic fold: therapeutic results and long-term follow-up. *Laryngoscope* 1995; 105: 734–746.

7. Mendenhall WM, Parsons JT, Devine JW *et al*. Squamous cell carcinoma of the pyriform sinus treated with surgery and/or radiotherapy. *Head Neck Surg* 1987; 10: 88–92.

8. Spector JG, Sessions DG, Emami B *et al*. Squamous cell carcinoma of the pyriform sinus: a nonrandomized comparison of therapeutic modalities and long term results. *Laryngoscope* 1995; 105: 397–406.

9. Vandenbrouck C, Sancho H, Lefur R *et al*. Results of a randomized clinical trial of preoperative irradiation versus postoperative irradiation in the treatment of tumors of the hypopharynx. *Cancer* 1977; 39: 1445–1449.

10. Marks JE, Kinnik B, Powers WE. Carcinoma of the pyriform sinus: an analysis of treatment results and patterns of failure. *Cancer* 1978; 41: 1008–1015.

11. Meoz-Mendez RT, Fletcher GH, Guillamondequi OM, Peters LJ. Analysis of the results of irradiation in the treatment of squamous cell carcinoma of the pharyngeal wall. *Int J Radiat Oncol Biol Phys* 1978; 4: 579–585.

12. Farrington WT, Weighall JS, Jones PH. Postcricoid carcinoma (a 10 year retrospective study). *J Laryngol Otol* 1986; 100: 79–84.

13. Pearson SG. Radiotherapy of carcinoma of the esophagus and postcricoid region in Southeast Scotland. *Clin Radiol* 1966; 17: 242–247.

14. Harrison DFN. Surgical repair of hypopharyngeal and cervical esophageal cancer. Analysis of 162 patients. *Ann Otol Rhinol Laryngol* 1981; 90: 372–375.

CHAPTER ten

Extent of resection of
hypopharyngeal cancer

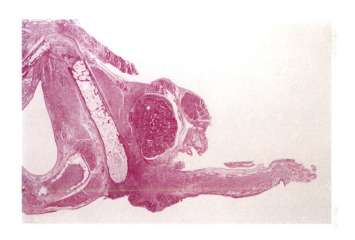

Introduction

Patients suffering from hypopharyngeal carcinoma frequently only seek medical treatment when they have significant symptoms. However, by this time, their disease is usually in late stage. Even for patients with advanced disease, surgery should be offered for all resectable cancers of the hypopharynx unless the patient declines surgical treatment or is medically unfit. The best outcome can be achieved for these patients when combined therapy is administered. This usually involves surgical resection followed by radiotherapy. Even when resection is not curative, surgery removes the primary tumour and relieves distressing dysphagia.

Surgical management comprises radical extirpation of the primary tumour together with the appropriate treatment of the cervical lymph nodes. The defect following surgical resection of the primary tumour should also be reconstructed so as to provide the patient with the best functional capability.

The nature of the surgical resection of the primary tumour depends on the condition of the patient, the surgical expertise available and, more importantly, the pathological extent of the tumour. Management of cervical lymph nodes may also affect outcome (Box 10.1).

Pathological behaviour

To date, the results of radical surgery for hypopharyngeal carcinoma have remained only fair. The 5-year survival rate following radical surgery and combined with radiotherapy ranges from 25% to 40% [1,2]. The main cause of failure is believed to be related to submucosal extension of the primary tumour. Our inability to recognize this leads to difficulty in determining the exact extent of resection, and this may give rise to local recurrence [3]. Pathological studies have shown that poor survival was associated with tumour in the cervical lymph nodes [4] and at the resection margins [5]. The presence of tumour in cervical lymph nodes is more frequent when the primary tumour is larger than 4 cm [5]. Adequate surgical resection can only be achieved with a knowledge of the pathological behaviour of hypopharyngeal carcinoma (Box 10.2).

Primary tumour

The presence of submucosal extension significantly affects the surgeon's ability to carry out adequate resection of the primary tumour. The extent of submucosal involvement measured from the edge of the tumour was found to be different when examined either superiorly and inferiorly, ranging from 10–20 mm and 10–30 mm, respectively [3,6,7]. Submucosal extension is not easy to detect clinically, and thus ample tissue must be removed beyond the tumour to achieve a curative resection. This results in quite extensive resection and major reconstruction which may in turn lead to increased morbidity and mortality.

A recent study of pathological specimens has revealed that the likelihood of submucosal extension in hypopharyngeal carcinoma is 58% [8]. Such extension can be classified into three types:

- Type I extension is manifest by a smooth tumour surface which elevates the mucosa, and is visible clinically (Fig. 10.1).
- Type II submucosal extension involves sheets of malignant cells that are located in the submucosa and not visualized on clinical examination (Fig. 10.2).
- Type III extension is a true skip lesion with healthy mucosa between the tumour nodules (Fig. 10.3).

Two-thirds of submucosal extensions are type I and the remaining one-third of patients have type II involvement, whereas type III is relatively uncommon. Type II submucosal extension is found significantly more frequently in patients who have received radiotherapy before surgery.

The spreads of submucosal extension in three directions, superiorly, laterally and inferiorly, were reported to be 3–10 mm, 2–37 mm and 3–35 mm, respectively. The presence of spread did not affect the tumour recurrence or survival, provided that a clear margin was achieved at surgical resection.

Although vertical and transverse spread of hypopharyngeal carcinoma is often extensive, deep extension is usually limited. Occasionally, hypopharyngeal carcinoma may extend anterolaterally to affect the thyroid cartilage, the strap muscles, and even the skin of the anterior neck. Posterior extension to the prevertebral muscles is very uncommon. Tumour sometimes infiltrates through the lateral wall to involve the sternomastoid muscle and

---

Box 10.1 *Factors influencing the extent of resection*

- Extent of primary tumour
- Surgical expertise available
- Extent of lymph node metastasis
- Patient's general and medical condition
- Aim of surgery, i.e. cure or palliation

Box 10.2 *Causes of failure in surgical treatment of hypopharyngeal carcinoma*

- Positive margin at resection
- Metastatic tumour spread to cervical lymph nodes
- Unrecognized submucosal spread

---

the internal jugular vein, but rarely affects the carotid vessels.

Cervical lymph nodes

Carcinoma of the hypopharynx has a notoriously high incidence of metastasis to the regional lymph nodes (Fig. 10.4). The likelihood of cervical lymph node metastasis depends on the location of the primary tumour and ranges from 40% to 75%, being most frequent when the primary carcinoma is in the piriform fossa [9–11]. When the primary tumour is close to the midline, then metastasis to the contralateral neck is not uncommon [12,13]. Retrospective studies of neck dissection specimens have shown that when lymph nodes in the neck are not palpable, then metastatic nodes were mostly located in level II and III. When lymph nodes were palpable in the neck, then metastatic nodes were found at all the levels [14]. The pattern of distribution of metastatic lymph nodes helps in planning surgical procedures.

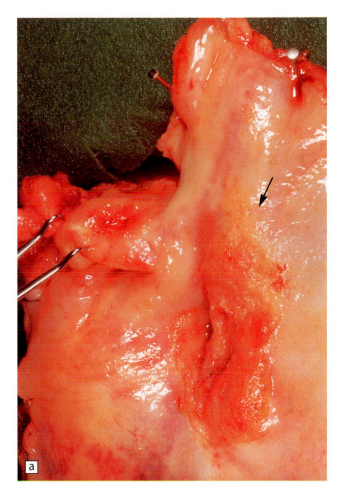

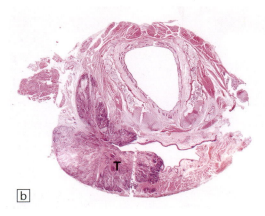

Figure 10.1 Type I submucosal tumour spread. (a) The submucosal tumour extension is seen as an elevation (arrow). (b) Histological section showing tumour (T) cells in the submucosa. (Haematoxylin & eosin staining; original magnification, × 80.)

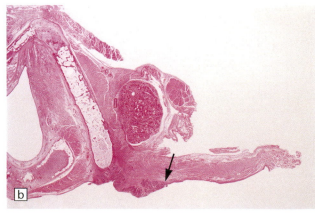

Figure 10.2 Type II submucosal tumour spread. (a) The submucosal tumour extension is not visible macroscopically (arrow). (b) Histological section showing tumour cells in the submucosa (arrow). (Haematoxylin & eosin staining; original magnification, × 80.)

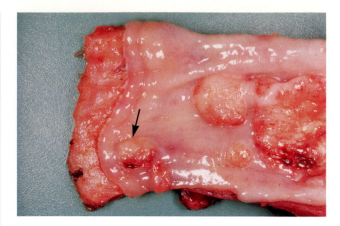

Figure 10.3 Type III submucosal tumour spread. Skip lesion (arrow) with intervening healthy mucosa.

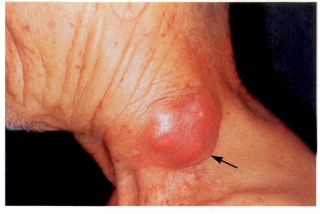

Figure 10.4 Clinical photograph showing a large metastatic cervical lymph node (arrow) in a patient suffering from carcinoma of hypopharynx.

Extent of resection

The aim of surgical resection of the primary lesion is to remove the tumour adequately so that resection margins are free of tumour. Pathological features of submucosal extension should be taken into account, and sufficient tissue removed to ensure all malignant disease is cleared. As for the cervical lymph nodes, the aim is to remove all the possible tumour-bearing areas with minimal morbidity.

Primary tumour

The size and shape of the hypopharynx is important in planning resection and subsequent reconstruction. The configuration of the hypopharynx is funnel-shaped, with a wide upper end and a narrow lower end. This transition of size is maintained by the skeleton of the hyoid and thyroid cartilages, which are larger from side to side in the upper part of the hypopharynx. The diameter of the lumen in the upper part of the opened hypopharyngeal wall can be twice as great as that of the lower portion (Fig. 10.5). When a specimen of hypopharynx is opened up from behind, it is quite obvious that the circumference of the pharyngeal wall is greater in its upper than its lower part. Thus, more pharyngeal wall is available following resection of tumour in the upper portion. The cervical oesophagus has an even smaller lumen and shorter circumference such that partial resection of the oesophageal wall is not practical. The cervical oesophagus descends into the mediastinum through a narrow thoracic inlet, and this technically limits the length of lower resection margin when a cervical approach is used above.

From information gained in the step serial pathological study of the resected specimens, recommended resection margins are 3 cm inferiorly and 2 cm both superiorly and laterally (Box 10.3). Patients with skip lesions should be identified by preoperative screening either endoscopically

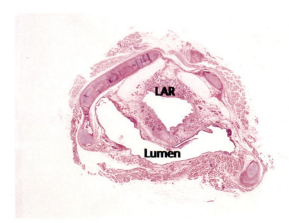

Figure 10.5 Histological section of the hypopharynx at the level of the vocal cords. The hypopharynx is a muscular tube (Lumen) with the larynx (LAR) as the anterior wall. (Haematoxylin & eosin staining; original magnification, × 80.)

Box 10.3 *Recommended resection margins*	
• Superior 2 cm	• Lateral 2 cm
• Inferior 3 cm	• Radial >1 mm

or with imaging studies and managed appropriately according to the distal extent of the skip lesion. For patients with visible (i.e. type I) submucosal extension, an adequate resection margin can achieved without too much difficulty. For type II submucosal extension – particularly in patients who have received previous radiotherapy – then a generous resection margin should be obtained at operation to ensure tumour clearance. Thus, depending on the location and extent of the main tumour, in addition to total laryngectomy, three types of resection of the hypopharynx may be considered.

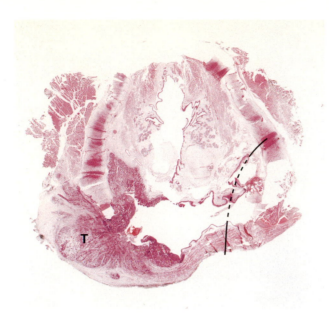

Figure 10.6 Histological section of the hypopharynx at the level of the larynx showing a tumour (T). Partial pharyngectomy can be carried out to remove tumour with adequate resection margin. The incision on the pharyngeal wall is marked (broken line). (Haematoxylin & eosin staining; original magnification, × 80.)

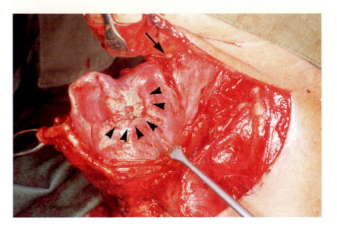

Figure 10.7 Intraoperative photograph with exposure of the hypopharyngeal carcinoma (arrowheads). This tumour can be removed with partial pharyngectomy. The incision over the pharynx (arrow) under direct vision ensures an adequate resection margin.

Partial pharyngectomy

For tumours located at a high level, e.g. the upper part of the piriform fossa unilaterally, it has often proved possible to remove the tumour with partial pharyngectomy and yet achieve an adequate resection margin (Figs 10.6, 10.7). This leaves a vertical strip of full-thickness pharyngeal wall lying between the oropharynx and the cervical oesophagus. The partial pharyngeal defect thus produced is not circumferential, but the width of the pharyngeal wall remaining is insufficient for direct closure, as performed following total laryngectomy (Fig. 10.8). Additional tissue is therefore required for reconstruction of the pharyngeal defect to facilitate swallowing.

Circumferential pharyngectomy

When the primary tumour occurs or extends to a lower level, such as the piriform fossa, the postcricoid region or the posterior wall, then the extent of resection should be carefully determined. At the lower part of the hypopharynx, the circumference narrows significantly, and removing the tumour with an adequate resection margin laterally on both sides will necessitate removal of the whole circumference of the hypopharynx (Fig. 10.9). Continuity of the hypopharynx is disrupted and there will be a circumferential defect between the oropharynx above and the cervical oesophagus below (Fig. 10.10). The

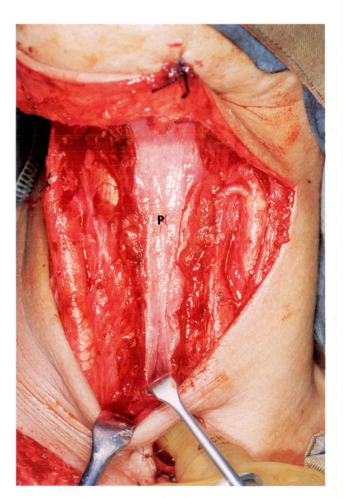

Figure 10.8 Intraoperative photograph showing the remaining pharyngeal mucosa after partial pharyngectomy. The narrow strip (P) cannot be tubed for reconstruction.

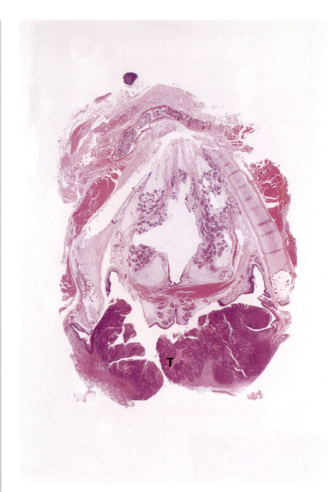

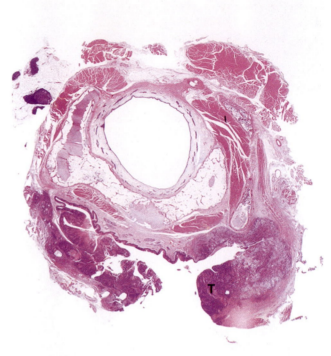

Figure 10.9 Histological section of the hypopharynx at the level of the arytenoids, showing a large tumour (T) arising from the posterior hypopharyngeal wall. Circumference is short, circumferential pharyngectomy is mandatory to ensure an adequate resection. (Haematoxylin & eosin staining; original magnification, × 80.)

Figure 10.11 Histological section of the hypopharynx at the level of postcricoid region, showing a tumour (T). To ensure adequate horizontal as well as vertical resection margins, the whole pharynx and oesophagus must be removed. (Haematoxylin & eosin staining; original magnification, × 80.)

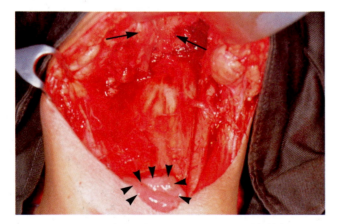

Figure 10.10 Intraoperative photograph showing the defect after circumferential pharyngectomy. The oropharyngeal opening is in the upper part (arrows), and the opening of the cervical oesophagus is below (arrowheads).

reconstruction method employed to restore continuity of the alimentary tract must bridge the defect.

Total pharyngolaryngo-oesophagectomy

For more inferiorly situated tumour, such as that arising from the lower postcricoid region, or hypopharyngeal carcinoma that has extended into the cervical oesophagus, then an augmented resection has to be performed (Fig. 10.11). The lumen of the cervical oesophagus is small, and adequate tumour clearance implies circumferential resection. Furthermore, as the cervical oesophagus measures only 5–6 cm in length, in order to achieve an adequate lower resection margin beyond the tumour, the line of transection of the oesophagus will need to be in the superior mediastinum.

On reconstruction, the lower anastomosis will be deep within the thoracic inlet down in the mediastinum.

Technically, it is difficult to achieve this with a superior approach alone, and any complication resulting from the anastomosis will be serious. An alternative procedure such as transhiatal total oesophagectomy may be carried out, being somewhat easier to reconstruct the resultant defect between the oropharynx and the cardia. When the stomach is mobilized and brought up through the posterior mediastinum for reconstruction, only one anastomosis – fashioned in the neck between the oropharynx and the gastric fundus – is required (Fig. 10.12).

The morbidity and mortality of resection and reconstruction are greater for pharyngolaryngo-oesophagectomy than for partial pharyngectomy [15]. Although tumour clearance is maximal with a more extensive resection, associated problems of a more radical operation are more likely.

Pharyngolaryngo-oesophagectomy has definite associated morbidity which may occur intraoperatively, such as bleeding or damage to the posterior tracheal wall [16]. Late complications are not negligible on long-term follow-up [17]. Although the risks associated with surgery have been reduced in recent years as a result of refinement of operative techniques, better preoperative preparation and patient selection [18], this operation should not be performed indiscriminately for all patients. The nature of the resection should be determined with the extent of primary tumour on an individual basis (Table 10.1).

Radial margin of clearance

The deep margin of resection of hypopharyngeal carcinoma is also important for tumour eradication. The prevertebral muscle, together with its overlying fascia, forms the posterior limit of tumour and these structures are rarely infiltrated even in advanced disease. Surgical clearance is frequently possible (Fig. 10.13).

The larynx forms an anterior barrier for hypopharyngeal carcinoma, and is removed *en bloc* at

pharyngeal resection. When a large tumour extends anterolaterally to involve the skin of the anterior neck, this should be removed for tumour clearance (Fig. 10.14). The resultant defect can be covered satisfactorily with a

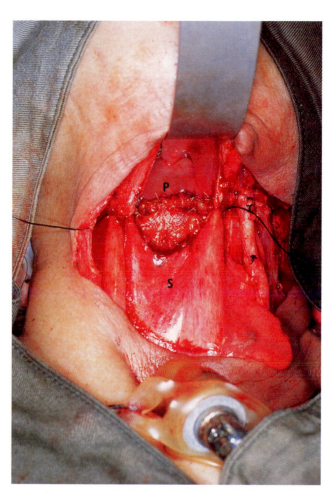

Figure 10.12 Intraoperative photograph. The stomach (S) was brought up through the posterior mediastinum and anastomosed to the pharynx (P).

Table 10.1 *Extent of resection in relation to extent of tumour*	
Location of tumour	**Extent of resection**
Upper part of hypopharynx, on one side	Partial pharyngectomy
Extensive tumour in upper hypopharynx Lower part of hypopharynx, not extending beyond postcricoid inferiorly	Circumferential pharyngectomy
Hypopharyngeal carcinoma extending into cervical oesophagus	Circumferential pharyngectomy + oesophagectomy

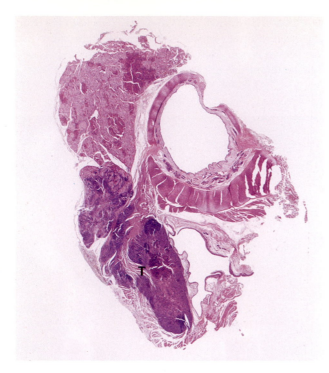

Figure 10.13 Histological section of the hypopharynx. The tumour (T) is well contained within the hypopharynx. Even though the deep resection margin is small, as long as it can be removed from the prevertebral fascia, tumour eradication is possible. (Haematoxylin & eosin staining; original magnification, × 80.)

regional flap (Fig. 10.15). When a myocutaneous flap or the stomach is used for reconstruction of the pharyngeal defect, then split thickness skin grafting over the muscle or the stomach has been successful in providing coverage (Fig. 10.16).

Lateral extension of the primary hypopharyngeal carcinoma to affect the sternomastoid muscle and the internal jugular vein is not uncommon when the primary tumour is large, and resection of these structures is mandatory for tumour extirpation. The carotid arterial wall is resistant to tumour invasion and can frequently be preserved. However, the external carotid artery may be encased by enlarged lymph nodes and it should be removed with the primary tumour. Resection of the common or internal carotid artery with a vascular replacement graft is not indicated, as no survival benefit is gained and associated morbidity may be substantial.

Cervical lymph nodes

In view of the high propensity of metastasis to cervical lymph nodes in patients suffering from hypopharyngeal carcinoma, attention to detail in the treatment of the lymph nodes is mandatory for curative therapy. The choice between radiotherapy or surgery depends on the treatment option employed for the primary lesion. When definitive radiotherapy is given, the neck should be included in the radiation field.

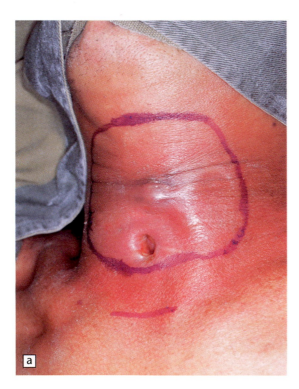

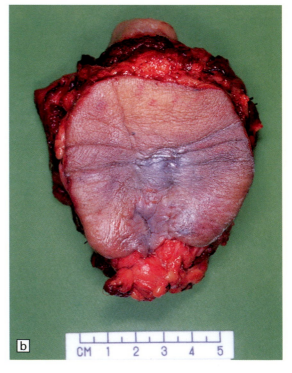

Figure 10.14 (a) When the anterior neck skin is involved, it should be removed with the laryngopharyngectomy. The incision is marked. (b) Specimen with anterior neck skin.

For patients with no palpable cervical lymph nodes, then selective neck dissection removing lymph nodes at levels II, III and IV should be performed *en bloc* with resection of the primary tumour as these are frequent sites of tumour metastasis. When cervical nodal metastasis can be palpated, then radical neck dissection should be carried out at pharyngectomy. For a primary tumour that crosses the midline, the contralateral neck should be managed, applying the same principles.

Summary

The ultimate aim in the management of hypopharyngeal carcinoma is to eradicate the tumour and to carry out appropriate reconstruction. The surgical option which causes minimal morbidity and allows the patient to retain maximal function should be chosen. This is dependent on the extent of the primary tumour, the status of the cervical lymph nodes, and also the surgical expertise available.

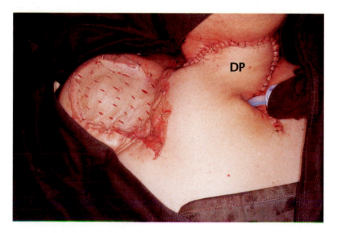

Figure 10.15 A deltopectoral flap (DP) is used to reconstruct the skin defect in the anterior neck.

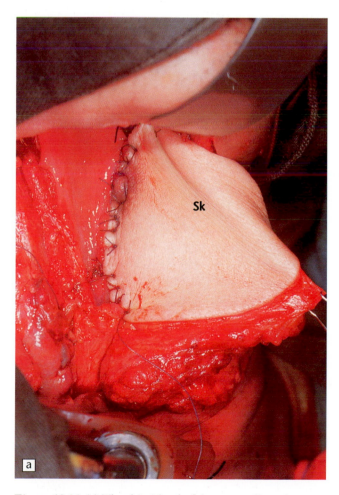

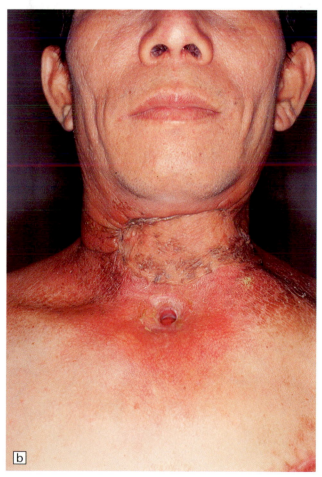

Figure 10.16 (a) The skin island of the pectoralis major myocutaneous flap (Sk) was employed to reconstruct the pharyngeal defect. The muscle bulk fills the defect in anterior neck. (b) Healed split thickness skin graft applied over the muscle for resurfacing the neck defect.

References

1. Shah JP, Shaha AR, Spiro RH, Strong EW. Carcinoma of the hypopharynx. *Am J Surg* 1976; 132: 439–443.

2. Kramer S, Gelber RD, Snow JB *et al*. Combined radiation therapy and surgery in the management of advanced head and neck cancer: final report of study 73-03 of the radiation therapy oncology group. *Head Neck Surg* 1987; 10: 19–30.

3. Harrison DFN. Pathology of hypopharyngeal cancer in relation to surgical management. *J Laryngol Otol* 1970; 84: 349–367.

4. Martin SA, Marks JE, Lee JY *et al*. Carcinoma of the pyriform sinus: predictors of TNM relapse and survival. *Cancer* 1980; 46: 1974–1981.

5. Sesions D. Surgical pathology of cancer of the larynx and hypopharynx. *Laryngoscope* 1976; 86: 814–819.

6. Hiroto I, Nomura Y, Sueyoshi K *et al*. Pathological studies related to neoplasms of the hypopharynx and cervical esophagus. *Kurume Med J* 1969; 16: 127–133.

7. Davidge-Pitts KJ, Mannel A. Pharyngolaryngectomy with extrathoracic esophagectomy. *Head Neck* 1983; 6: 571–574.

8. Ho CM, Ng WF, Lam KH *et al*. Submucosal tumor extension in hypopharyngeal cancer. *Arch Otolaryngol Head Neck Surg* 1997; 123: 959–965.

9. Hahn SS, Spaulding CA, Kim JA, Constable WC. The prognostic significance of lymph node involvement in pyriform sinus and supraglottic cancers. *Int J Radiat Oncol Biol Phys* 1987; 13: 1143–1147.

10. Lefebvre JL, Castelain B, De La Torre JC *et al*. Lymph node invasion in hypopharynx and lateral epilarynx carcinoma: a prognostic factor. *Head Neck Surg* 1987; 10: 14–18.

11. Ballantyne AJ. Methods of repair after surgery for cancer of the pharyngeal wall, postcricoid area and cervical esophagus. *Am J Surg* 1971; 122: 482–486.

12. Byers RM, Wolf PF, Ballantyne AJ. Rationale for elective modified neck dissection. *Head Neck Surg* 1988; 10: 160–167.

13. Guillamondegui OM, Meoz R, Jesse RH. Surgical treatment of squamous cell carcinoma of the pharyngeal walls. *Am J Surg* 1978; 136: 474–476.

14. Candela FC, Kothari K, Shah JP. Patterns of cervical node metastases from squamous carcinoma of the oropharynx and hypopharynx. *Head Neck Surg* 1990; 12: 197–203.

15. Ho CM, Lam KH, Wei WI *et al*. Squamous cell carcinoma of the hypopharynx – analysis of treatment results. *Head Neck* 1993; 15: 405–412.

16. Wei WI, Lam KH, Lau WF *et al*. Salvageable mediastinal problems in pharyngolaryngo-esophagectomy and pharyngogastric anastomosis. *Head Neck Surg* 1988; 10: S60–S68.

17. Wei WI, Lam KH, Choi S, Wong J. Late problems after pharyngolaryngoesophagectomy and pharyngogastric anastomosis for cancer of the larynx and hypopharynx. *Am J Surg* 1984; 148: 509–513.

18. Lam KH, Choi TK, Wei WI *et al*. Present status of pharyngogastric anastomosis following pharyngolaryngo-oesophagectomy. *Br J Surg* 1987; 74: 122–125.

CHAPTER eleven

Reconstruction of the hypopharynx

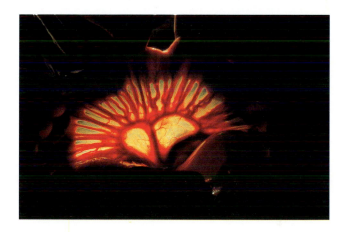

Introduction

After adequate extirpation of the tumour in the hypopharynx, the defect thus created should be reconstructed appropriately to provide optimal function. Local cervical skin flaps were first employed 30 years ago for reconstruction of the defect following pharyngolaryngectomy [1]. Reconstruction must be carried out in stages, and the whole procedure requires 4–6 months for completion. Even when reconstruction has been successful, the ability to swallow has been limited by the stenosis which frequently occurs at the mucocutaneous junction.

In recent years, with more advanced techniques, reconstruction of the hypopharyngeal defect is nearly always performed at the time of the resection [2]. Frequently, tissues outside radiation fields are used and the choice of reconstructive methods adopted depends on a number of factors such as the three-dimensional configuration of the defect, the patient's condition, and the surgical expertise available. The reliability of individual reconstructive options and the functional ability produced are additional concerns. Needless to say, the procedure employed for the patient should have minimal morbidity [3] (Box 11.1).

Reconstruction

Following the resection of hypopharyngeal carcinoma, as described in Chapter 10, one of three types of defect will result. The choice of method of reconstruction depends on the nature of the defect created after adequate surgical resection of the hypopharyngeal tumour [4]. The reconstructive options for each defect are outlined below.

Partial pharyngeal defect

This is the resultant defect following partial pharyngectomy. Essentially, the posterior pharyngeal wall is retained and continues as the posterior wall of the cervical oesophagus. The integrity of the alimentary tract can be reconstituted with a patch of epithelial-lined tissue. The options for reconstruction include free flaps and pedicle flaps. The latter are used frequently as they are relatively simple to raise and inset. The pedicle flaps are reliable, and the donor site is usually outside the radiation field. Free flaps are not used as a first choice for this type of defect as the recipient vessels in the neck may be removed when a radical neck dissection is carried out, together with resection of the primary tumour. Although requiring particular surgical expertise, the functional results of reconstruction with a free flap are not better than those obtained with a pedicled flap (Table 11.1).

Deltopectoral flaps, although reliable and easy to harvest, are not currently in frequent use. Their application requires the creation of a temporary salivary fistula, the closure of which then requires a secondary procedure to be performed. Myocutaneous flaps, such as

---

> **Box 11.1** *Factors influencing the choice of reconstruction options*
>
> - Extent of defect created after resection
> - Expected results of the reconstruction, both function and form
> - General condition of the patient
> - Surgical expertise available
> - Previous radiotherapy

Table 11.1 *Factors affecting the choice of flaps for partial pharyngeal defect*

	Pedicled myocutaneous flap	Free flap
One-stage operation	Yes	Yes
Donor site outside radiation field	Yes	Yes
Preparation in the neck	Neck dissection required to create space for myocutaneous flap	Recipient vessels preparation mandatory
Donor site morbidity	Minimal	Minimal
Surgical expertise	Yes	Very much
Functional results	Good	Good

the pectoralis major or the latissimus dorsi myocutaneous flaps, are proving to be the most popular. Reconstruction with a pectoralis major myocutaneous flap can be carried out with the patient in the same position as that adopted for resection, whereas a latissimus dorsi flap requires a change of position. A latissimus dorsi flap provides a better cosmetic result at the donor site, though this may not be of great importance in patients suffering from hypopharyngeal carcinoma.

When a myocutaneous flap with a skin island is used for reconstruction of the partial pharyngeal defect, a neck dissection is usually carried out at the same time. Removal of the sternomastoid muscle is necessary to create space to accommodate the bulk of the myocutaneous flap. As this muscle bulk will make subsequent palpation of the neck nodes difficult, lymph nodes in the neck are usually removed.

Surgical procedure

The size of the defect is measured and a comparable skin island is marked on the anterior chest wall over the pectoralis major myocutaneous flap. In general, the skin will contract in size by approximately 10% in both directions after incision. This must be taken into account when planning reconstruction so as to avoid subsequent stretching which may jeopardize the blood supply to the skin island. As there are more musculocutaneous perforating vessels laterally, the skin island should be placed as laterally as possible. The skin island should be situated entirely over the pectoralis major muscle to ensure that it is nourished by all the perforators from the muscle (Box 11.2).

The pectoral branch of the acromiothoracic trunk which supplies the pectoralis major myocutaneous flap descends on the undersurface of the muscle. The vascular pedicle is identified in the groove between the clavicular and the sternocostal portions of the pectoralis major myocutaneous flap. The latter portion alone is adequate to carry the skin island and, thus, the clavicular head of the muscle can be divided to allow the pedicle to be moved up smoothly (Fig. 11.1). The thin pedicle lying over the clavicle is not distorted by any muscle bulk and is more mobile. All these manoeuvres contribute to the elimination of tension of the vascular pedicle and thus to improved viability of the flap [5].

The epithelial surface of the skin island when transposed to the neck will be facing inwards, and this is sutured to the pharyngeal wall with interrupted sutures. Postoperatively, oral feeding is resumed when imaging studies – such as barium swallow – show complete healing of the pharyngeal wound. Myocutaneous flaps are reliable, and their application for the reconstruction of this type of defect has a high success rate with satisfactory preservation of swallowing function.

> **Box 11.2** *Essential points on raising the pectoralis major myocutaneous flap*
>
> - Whole skin island should be lying on the pectoralis major muscle
> - The planned skin island should be 10% larger than the defect to allow shrinkage
> - The skin island should be planned to be over the lateral aspect of the pectoralis major muscle where there are more perforators
> - The sternocostal portion of the muscle alone is adequate to support the skin island

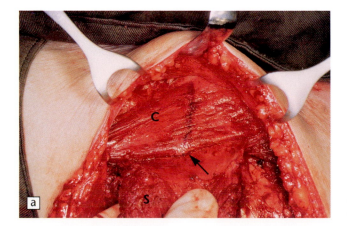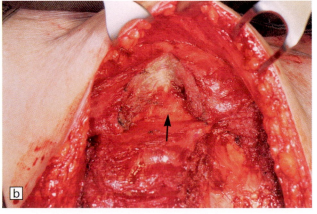

Figure 11.1 (a) Intraoperative photograph showing that the sternocostal portion (S) is separated from the clavicular portion (C) of the pectoralis major muscle. The incision over the clavicular portion is marked (arrow). (b) The clavicular portion of the muscle is divided, and the muscle fibres retracted to provide a gap (arrow) for the pedicle of the flap once it is turned upwards for pharyngeal reconstruction.

Circumferential pharyngeal defect

The defect following a circumferential pharyngectomy is more challenging as continuity of the alimentary tract is lost and reconstruction can be more problematic. The gap between the oropharynx above and the cervical oesophagus below needs to be reconstructed. Stricture of the circular anastomoses both at the upper and the lower margins must be avoided, and swallowing restored. The options for reconstruction are the use of myocutaneous flaps or free flaps which can be either be in the form of a free jejunal graft or a radial forearm flap sutured as a skin tube.

Myocutaneous flaps

When a pectoralis major myocutaneous flap is employed, the design of the skin island is important. The defect should be accurately measured and the length of the skin island marked out accordingly. Besides taking into account the expected 10% shrinkage in size, it should be at least 2 cm longer than the defect as there will be a loss in length when the interdigitating suturing method is employed for the upper and lower circular anastomoses. The width of the skin island should be at least 6 cm in order to provide a reconstructed skin tube with a 2 cm diameter. The skin island is usually longer than that employed for repairing a partial pharyngeal defect. Although it is wiser to place the skin island as laterally as possible where there are more musculocutaneous perforators, it is usually positioned to the medial side of the nipple so that its entire length overlies the pectoralis major muscle. The shape of the skin island should be in the form of a trapezium, with the shorter edge on its upper part. This upper edge of the skin island, when transposed to the neck, will be anastomosed to the cervical oesophagus which is narrower than the oropharynx (Box 11.3).

The skin island of the myocutaneous flap is fashioned into a tube and then anastomosed to the oropharynx above and cervical oesophagus below. To prevent stricture formation – which is not uncommon for circular anastomoses between mucocutaneous junctions – the anastomosis is carried out in a fashion to avoid a circular suture line. Three incisions are made separately over the oropharynx and the cervical oesophagus, splitting them into three segments. Similar incisions are made over the skin island (Fig. 11.2) so that at anastomosis, skin island flaps can be sutured in an interdigitating fashion with the corresponding flaps from the oropharynx and the cervical oesophagus [6] (Figs 11.3, 11.4). In this way, the suture line is in a wave-like form rather than circular. On healing, the scarring stretches the anastomosis wider rather than causing it to stenose.

A tubed skin island of myocutaneous flap is a reliable method for reconstruction of circumferential defects. In obese patients, however, it is technically difficult to suture a thick piece of skin into a tube, and suturing will create 'T' junctions at the upper and lower anastomoses. The incidence of leakage is significant and although the fistula usually heals eventually with conservative treatment,

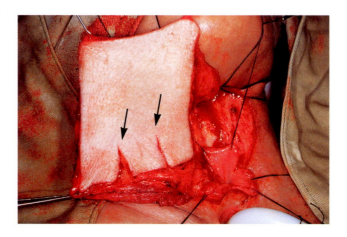

Figure 11.2 Intraoperative photograph showing the incisions (arrows) over the skin island of the pectoralis major myocutaneous flap for interdigitating suturing.

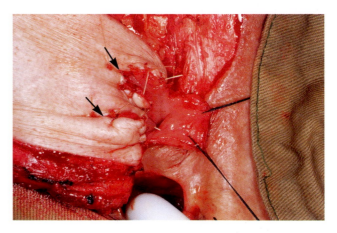

Figure 11.3 Intraoperative photograph showing the incisions over the cervical oesophagus allowing interdigitating suturing of the mucocutaneous junction (arrows).

Box 11.3 *Essential points for raising the pectoralis major myocutaneous flap for reconstruction of a circumferential pharyngeal defect*

- The skin island should be placed more medially so that it lies entirely on the pectoralis major muscle
- The skin island should be 2 cm longer than the vertical pharyngeal defect to allow interdigitating suturing
- The width of the skin island should be 6 cm or more
- The skin island should be trapezium-shaped to accommodate the pharyngeal defect

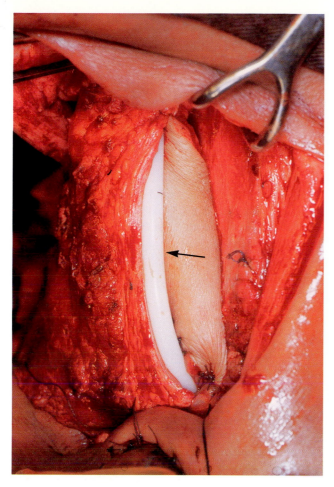

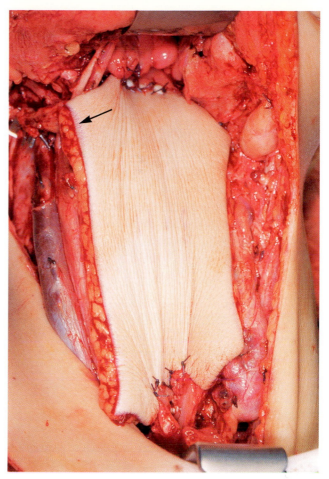

Figure 11.4 After similar procedures carried out on the oropharyngeal end, the skin island is gradually turned into a tube. A nasogastric tube is placed within the lumen (arrow).

Figure 11.5 The radial forearm cutaneous flap is used for reconstruction of circumferential pharyngeal defect. Interdigitating suturing is employed. The vascular pedicle is shown (arrow).

prolonged periods of convalescence may be required. Swallowing is usually adequate when the pharyngeal segment is reconstructed with a skin tube; however, this technique is regarded as being inferior when compared with other methods of reconstruction.

Free flaps

Radial forearm flap

The radial forearm skin island can be used to reconstruct a circumferential pharyngeal defect by tubing the skin island. The radial forearm skin is hairless and thin, and easier to suture into a tube to bridge the gap between the oropharynx and the cervical oesophagus. Its limitations are the increased incidence of stricture formation at the mucocutaneous junction, and swallowing is inferior. This complication can be reduced when the interdigitating suturing method is employed (Fig. 11.5). With this method of reconstruction, a skin surface is used to line the alimentary tract and without the secretion of

mucus – as happens in bowel – the passage of food material is slow.

Jejunum

Currently, the most frequently used method for reconstruction of a circumferential defect of the hypopharynx is the transposition of a segment of jejunum from the abdomen to the neck. The blood supply of the jejunum can be reconstituted by anastomosis of the jejunal vessels with the appropriate vessels in the neck. Usually, the second vascular arcade from the ligament of Treiz is used, as at this site the vessels are relatively straight with a size comparable with that of the recipient vessels in the neck (Fig. 11.6). The vascular anastomosis is performed under magnification with interrupted sutures. Any suitable branch from the external carotid artery can be used as the recipient artery, and the jejunal vein is usually joined to a branch of the internal jugular vein. The size of the jejunal lumen is comparable with that of the cervical oesophagus, and an end-to-end anastomosis can usually be accomplished comfortably. The discrepancy in size between the jejunum and the oropharynx at the upper anastomosis can be handled by slitting the jejunal wall at the antimesenteric border so that a longer circumference is made available for anastomosis.

Although the likelihood of failure of a free jejunal graft is generally believed to be approximately 10%, mostly being attributed to various problems of the vascular pedicle, with more practice the success rate has increased in recent years to over 95% (Fig. 11.7). Once the free jejunal graft reconstruction is successful, the patient can resume normal diet within a week of operation. The incidence of fistula formation and stricture are low when the bowel anastomosis is carried out satisfactorily. In view of the extensive nature of the primary tumour, post-operative radiotherapy is usually given to the tumour bed. This radiation field usually includes the whole graft, but morbidity related to the jejunum following radiotherapy is, fortunately, rare. Initially, the mucosa may show some reactive changes which recover after 3 months. However, submucosal fibrosis and loss of glands may persist for years after completion of radiotherapy [7] (Figs 11.8, 11.9).

In order to carry out a successful free jejunal graft expeditiously, one surgical team should harvest a segment of jejunum, while another team is carrying out the resection and preparing the recipient vessels in the neck. The jejuno-oesophageal anastomosis is usually performed before the microvascular anastomosis. This allows the fixation of the bowel to a certain extent to avoid excessive traction on the vascular pedicle. The microvascular anastomosis of artery and vein are carried out with the operating microscope for magnification. Finally, the upper anastomosis between the oropharynx and the jejunum is sutured. The cold ischaemic time of the jejunum is less than 2–3 h; thus, the entire procedure of free jejunal

grafting should be completed within this time to ensure viability. Postoperatively, the free jejunal graft can be monitored by flexible endoscopic examination whenever indicated (Fig. 11.10).

Currently, when the surgical expertise is available, a free jejunal graft is the optimal reconstruction method for circumferential pharyngeal defects (Table 11.2).

Laryngopharyngo-oesophageal defect

When the primary tumour in the hypopharynx is extensive and adequate tumour clearance can only be achieved with total pharyngolaryngo-oesophagectomy, then the defect is extensive. This can be reconstructed by mobilizing the stomach and transposing it through the posterior mediastinum to be anastomosed to the oropharynx.

This operation was first introduced in 1960 and has gained popularity world-wide as both resection and re-construction can be carried out in one stage. In addition, there is only one anastomosis between the oropharynx and the stomach [8]. The hospital mortality associated with the operation was high in the 1970s [9,10], but with improved surgical technique and patient support measures this has been much reduced in recent years [11–13].

Surgical technique

After mobilizing the larynx and the hypopharynx with the primary tumour, the oesophagus is mobilized from the neck down into the mediastinum, taking care not to damage the posterior tracheal wall (Fig. 11.11). Deflation of the cuff of the tracheostomy tube during this procedure is helpful. Laparotomy is undertaken and the lower part of the oesophagus is mobilized transhiatally. After dividing the cardia, the specimen is delivered through the neck. The cardia is closed and the stomach is fashioned into a tube form with the fundus at one end (Fig. 11.12). The

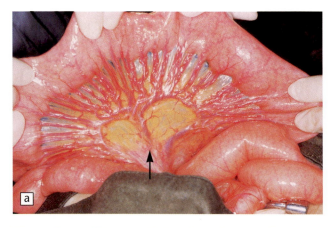
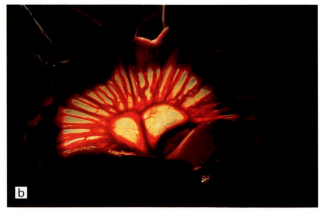

Figure 11.6 (a) The second jejunal vessel (arrow) from the ligament of Treiz is usually straight and supplies the appropriate length of jejunum. (b) The same segment of jejunum with the light shining from the back for a better delineation of the vascular pattern.

blood supply of the stomach is maintained from the right gastric and right gastroepiploic vessels. A pyloromyotomy is carried out to reduce postoperative gastric stasis (Fig. 11.13). A rubber tube is delivered from the hiatus to the neck. The lower end of the tube is sutured to the fundus of the stomach. By gently pulling the tube in the neck and pushing from below, the stomach is delivered to the neck through the posterior mediastinum.

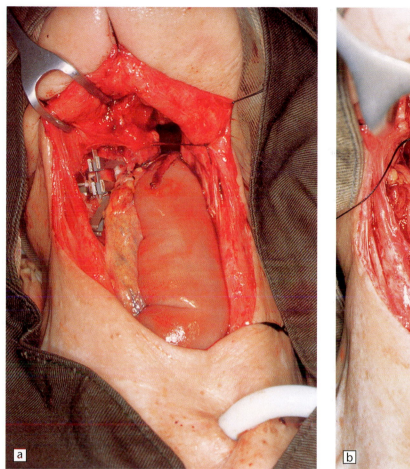

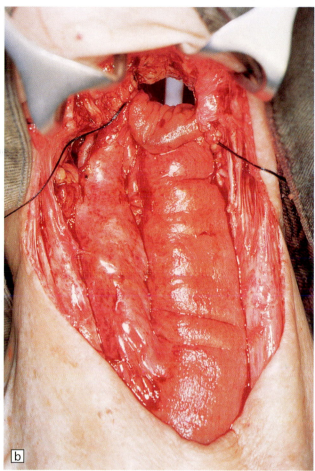

Figure 11.7 The free jejunal graft in position. The lower jejuno-oesophageal anastomosis is performed first, followed by the microvascular anastomosis. (a) Before releasing the vascular clamps. (b) After releasing the clamps, the jejunum is revascularized and the upper anastomosis can be carried out at leisure.

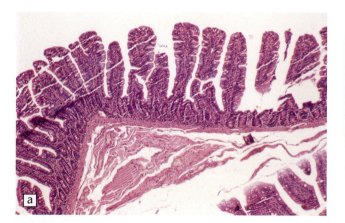

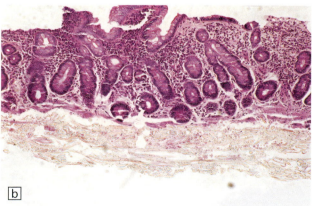

Figure 11.8 Histological slides of (a) normal jejunal mucosa and (b) jejunal mucosa after radiotherapy, showing atrophy of the villi.

Table 11.2 *Comparing the three options of reconstruction of circumferential pharyngeal defects*

	Tubed patch myocutaneous flap	Tubed radial forearm free flap	Free jejunal graft
Surgical reconstruction	Difficult to suture into a tube, especially with thick chest wall skin	Forearm skin is thin, easy to suture into a tube	Anastomosis to pharynx and oesophagus not difficult
Donor site	Chest wall defect can be closed primarily	Forearm defect repair requires skin graft	Primary anastomosis of jejunum
Complication	Stenosis at mucocutaneous junction frequent	Stenosis at mucocutaneous junction possible	Stenosis at anastomosis infrequent
Swallowing function	Fair, as skin is thick and may have hair	Good, as the skin is thin and hairless	Excellent, as lubricated by jejunal secretion

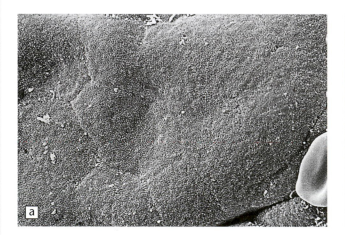
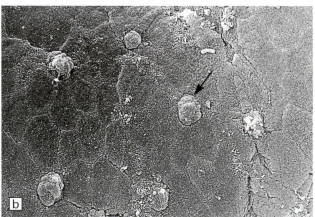

Figure 11.9 Scanning election microscopy of (a) normal jejunal mucosa and (b) jejunal mucosa after radiotherapy, showing atrophy of the mucosa, making the globlet cells more prominent (arrow).

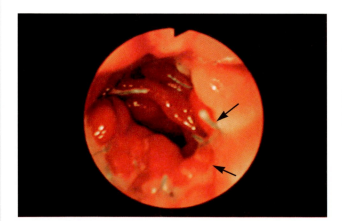

Figure 11.10 Early postoperative endoscopic view of the pharyngojejunal anastomosis, showing a viable jejunum. The suture line with stitches is indicated (arrows).

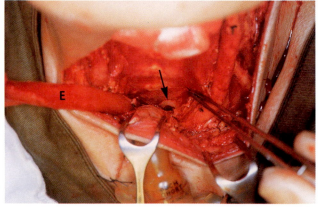

Figure 11.11 Intraoperative photograph viewing from the neck downwards. The tumour in the hypopharynx is wrapped up and blunt dissection is carried out around the oesophagus (E) down into the posterior mediastinum. The thoracic duct coming up from the posterior is seen (arrow).

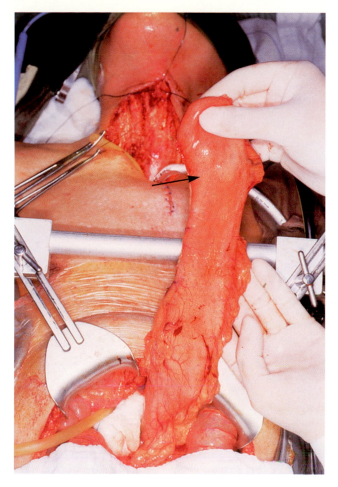

Figure 11.12 The cardia of the stomach is closed (arrow) and the stomach is fashioned into a tube form for delivery through the posterior mediastinum up to the neck.

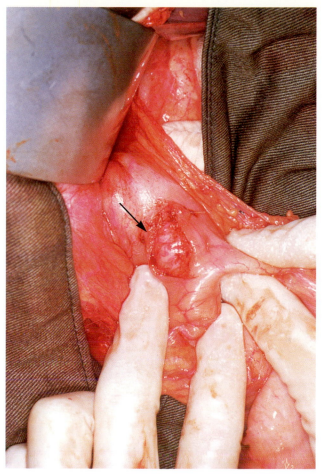

Figure 11.13 A pyloromyotomy is performed to reduce postoperative gastric stasis. After dividing the circular muscle fibres at the pylorus, the bulging mucosa can be seen (arrow).

Pharyngogastric anastomosis is then carried out with interrupted sutures. The posterior wall is sutured to the fundus of the stomach and the anterior wall of the stomach is incised in a 'T'-shaped incision (Fig. 11.14). This allows the anterior wall of the stomach to move up to the lateral aspects of the anastomosis, and the tongue base can be brought down to be sutured to the anterior stomach wall. All these manoeuvres help to reduce tension at the anastomosis for optimal healing.

Even though hospital mortality has decreased during recent years, the operation is associated with a certain degree of morbidity [14]. Many patients present with the disease at an advanced stage and are undernourished. Moreover, they are usually debilitated and are chronic smokers. The operative procedure involves three compartments of the body, and the consequences of surgical trauma are substantial. To reduce the mortality and morbidity, patients should be nourished before operation

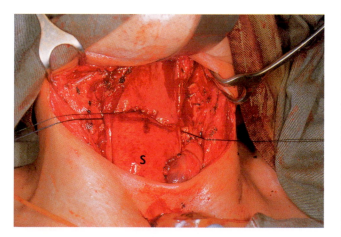

Figure 11.14 The stomach delivered to the neck. The incision over the anterior stomach (S) is made in a 'T' fashion. This allows the anterior wall of the stomach to move up laterally to reduce tension at the anastomosis.

with parenteral nutrition. The surgical trauma should be minimized as much as possible. The blunt dissection manoeuvre to mobilize the oesophagus in the posterior mediastinum transhiatally from below and transcervically from above can now be achieved with thoracoscope-assisted dissection intrathoracically. This may help to reduce surgical trauma and thus postoperative pulmonary complications (Box 11.4).

When performed judiciously, this operation – even in patients with advanced disease – invariably relieves the distressing symptom of dysphagia. In addition, the long-term effect of transposing the stomach to the neck does not greatly affect the well-being of the patient [15]. In selected patients, it is the operation of choice for reconstruction of the defect created by pharyngolaryngo-oesophagectomy.

Summary

Decisions regarding reconstruction options of the pharyngeal defect after adequate tumour ablation depend mainly on the extent of the defect. The patched myocutaneous flap should be employed for a partial pharyngeal defect, while a microvascular free jejunal graft is preferred for circumferential loss. When a pharyngolaryngo-oesophagectomy is carried out, then the defect can best be reconstructed by mobilizing the stomach to the neck pharyngogastric anastomosis. The reconstruction procedure which carries the least mortality and morbidity should be used. Moreover, it is important that the choice of the reconstruction procedure only be made following resection. Adequate tumour ablation is essential in the treatment of hypopharyngeal carcinoma, and resection should not be influenced by the availability of certain reconstruction techniques (Box 11.5).

Box 11.4 *Measures to reduce morbidity and mortality of gastric transposition*

- Patient selection
- Nutritional support for patients before operation
- Thoracoscopic mobilization of oesophagus under direct vision
- Reduce tension at pharyngogastric anastomosis

Box 11.5 *Reconstruction of pharyngeal defect: salient points*

- Adequate tumour extirpation is essential
- Reconstruction follows resection

Partial pharyngectomy	Patch myocutaneous flap
Circumferential pharyngectomy	Free jejunal graft
Pharyngo-oesophagectomy	Gastric transposition

References

1. Wookey H. The surgical treatment of carcinoma of the hypopharynx and the oesophagus. *Br J Surg* 1948; 35: 249–266.

2. Surkin MI, Lawson W, Biller HF. Analysis of the methods of pharyngoesophageal reconstruction. *Head Neck Surg* 1984; 6: 953–970.

3. Lau WF, Lam KH, Wei WI. Reconstruction of hypopharyngeal defects in cancer surgery: do we have a choice? *Am J Surg* 1987; 154: 374–380.

4. Lam KH, Lau WF, Wei WI. Tumor clearance at resection margins in total laryngectomy – a clinicopathologic study. *Cancer* 1988; 61: 2260–2272.

5. Wei WI, Lam KH, Wong J. The true pectoralis major myocutaneous island flap: an anatomical study. *Br J Plast Surg* 1984; 37: 568–573.

6. Lam KH, Wei WI, Lau WF. Avoiding stenosis in the tubed greater pectoral flap in pharyngeal repair. *Arch Otolaryngol Head Neck Surg* 1987; 113: 428–431.

7. Wei WI, Lam LK, Yuen PW *et al*. Mucosal changes of the free jejunal graft in response to radiotherapy. *Am J Surg* 1998; 175: 44–46.

8. Ong GB, Lee TC. Pharyngogastric anastomosis after oesophago-pharyngectomy for carcinoma of the hypopharynx and cervical oesophagus. *Br J Surg* 1960; 48: 193–200.

9. Spiro RH, Shah JP, Strong EW *et al*. Gastric transposition in head and neck surgery. *Am J Surg* 1983; 146: 483–487.

10. Lam KH, Wong J, Lim STK, Ong GB. Pharyngogastric anastomosis following pharyngolaryngoesophagectomy. Analysis of 157 cases. *World J Surg* 1981; 5: 509–516.

11. Cahow CE, Sasaki CT. Gastric pull-up reconstruction for pharyngo-laryngo-esophagectomy. *Arch Surg* 1994; 129: 425–430.

12. Lam KH, Choi TK, Wei WI *et al*. Present status of pharyngogastric anastomosis following pharyngolaryngo-oesophagectomy. *Br J Surg* 1987; 74: 122–125.

13. Marmuse J, Koka VN, Guedon C, Benhamou G. Surgical treatment of carcinoma of the proximal esophagus. *Am J Surg* 1995; 169: 386–390.

14. Wei WI. Current status of pharyngolaryngo-oesophagectomy and pharyngogastric anastomosis. *Head Neck* 1998; 20: 240–244.

15. Wei WI, Lam KH, Choi S, Wong J. Late problems after pharyngolaryngoesophagectomy and pharyngogastric anastomosis for cancer of the larynx and hypopharynx. *Am J Surg* 1984; 148: 509–513.

CHAPTER twelve

Complications of
surgical management of
hypopharyngeal cancer

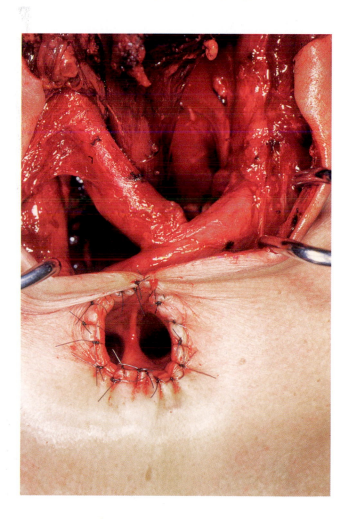

Introduction

Complications associated with the surgical management of hypopharyngeal cancer may occur either during the operation or in the postoperative period. The problems may be grouped in relation to the procedures of resection or reconstruction. Early recognition and proper management of these complications is mandatory in order to achieve a successful therapeutic outcome for the patient. On many occasions, complications may be avoided by taking appropriate precautions during the initial operation. The timing of correct management with regard to any particular problem is also important if a favourable outcome is to be achieved (Table 12.1).

Resection-related problems

Intraoperative problems

Bleeding

The occurrence of bleeding during the resection of hypopharyngeal carcinoma can usually be controlled easily, as the operative field in the neck is widely exposed.

When the carotid arterial system is injured, small holes may be repaired directly with sutures after controlling the proximal and distal ends of the artery. More extensive damage of the arterial wall can be similarly repaired with a venous patch. The external carotid artery can be ligated without sequelae. When a segment of the internal carotid artery must be removed because of either tumour infiltration or iatrogenic damage, then reconstruction can be achieved with direct anastomosis of the divided vessel after mobilization (Fig. 12.1). When there is loss of vascular tissue, then segmental interposition of a saphenous vein graft or a synthetic graft is necessary to restore arterial supply to the brain. The risk of hypoxic damage of the brain depends on the age of the patient, the collateral circulation, and also the duration of arterial occlusion.

The problem is more serious when intrathoracic bleeding occurs during blunt mobilization of the oesophagus. The small oesophageal vessels usually do not cause any problem, but if the azygos vein is injured, the bleeding can be torrential. It is difficult to control the bleeding by direct pressure on the torn vessel, as the damaged segment is in the thoracic cavity. The patient's blood pressure will drop very quickly, and unless immediate remedial measures are instituted, the patient will die from exsanguination. The anaesthetist should be alerted and volume replacement with blood or plasma expander should be administered immediately and rapidly to maintain a reasonable blood pressure.

The vertical upper abdominal incision should be extended immediately upwards to continue into a right anterior thoracotomy incision (Fig. 12.2). The right lung should be retracted anteriorly to allow identification of the damaged azygos vein and to institute haemostasis. Once the thorax is opened, the control of bleeding is not difficult and the situation can usually be salvaged (Fig. 12.3). The decision to perform an immediate thoracotomy is mandatory for the successful management of

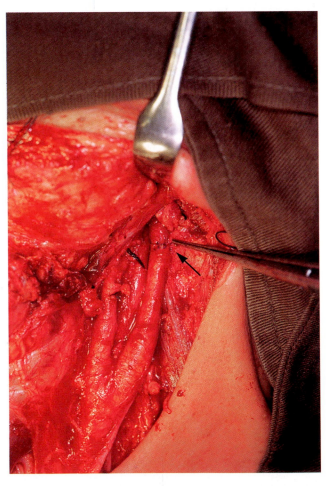

Figure 12.1 Intraoperative photograph. After removing a short segment of the internal carotid artery during neck dissection because of tumour involvement, the continuity of the vessel is restored with an end-to-end anastomosis (arrow).

Table 12.1 *Complications of surgical management of hypopharyngeal cancer*

Intraoperative	Postoperative
Bleeding in neck	Dehiscence of repair
Bleeding in mediastinum	Chylous fistula
Damage of tracheal wall	Recurrence
Perforations in gastrointestinal tract	

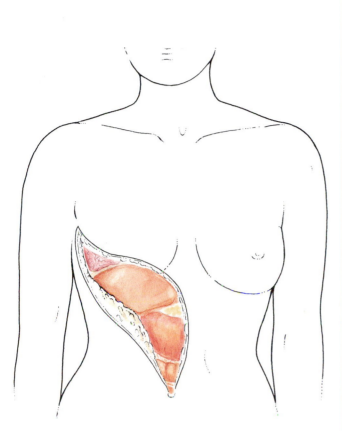

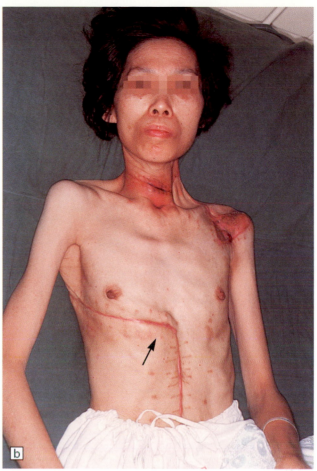

Figure 12.2 (a) Schematic drawing showing the extension of the upper midline abdominal incision to an anterior thoracotomy. (b) A patient who survived the operation, showing the incision (arrow).

these serious bleeding complications. In recent years, with the application of thoracoscopic assistance in the mobilization of the oesophagus, the azygos vein is dissected under direct vision so that this complication may be avoided [1].

Damage of the internal jugular vein in the neck can also be secured with direct suturing when both the upper and lower ends of the vessel are controlled. When the venous end retracts either upwards into the skull base or downwards into the mediastinum, then haemostasis may be difficult.

When the upper end of the internal jugular vein retracts and continues to bleed, temporary control of bleeding can be achieved with pressure, and adequate exposure should be gained for complete haemostasis. The digastric muscle can be retracted or divided to allow the application of clamps or sutures. On occasion, a mandibulotomy may even be necessary to expose the skull base to secure complete control of the bleeding vessel end. When the divided lower end of the internal jugular vein retracts into the upper thorax, in addition to applying

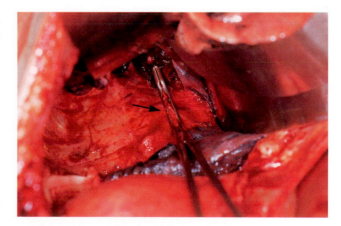

Figure 12.3 Intraoperative photograph showing the application of a vascular clamp (arrow) on the injured azygos vein to achieve haemostasis after the anterior thoracotomy.

pressure to gain temporary control of bleeding, the patient should be placed in the Trendelenburg position to avoid air being sucked into the large intrathoracic veins. When control of bleeding is not possible from the neck, it is much safer to split the sternum, after which the venous stump can be controlled in the upper chest (Fig. 12.4). In this way, correct haemostasis can be achieved safely (Table 12.2).

Damage of the post-tracheal wall

Injury of the posterior tracheal wall may occur during separation of the posterior tracheal wall from the upper part of the oesophagus. This is particularly so when the hypopharyngeal tumour extends into the cervical oesophagus and becomes adherent to the posterior tracheal wall (Fig. 12.5). The balloon of the endotracheal tube or the tracheostomy tube should be deflated to reduce the distension of the posterior tracheal wall during its separation from the oesophagus. When the posterior tracheal wall is damaged in the upper portion of the trachea, it can be repaired from the neck wound (Fig. 12.6). When direct repair cannot be carried out from the neck, then the associated morbidity is significant.

Injury of the lower part of the trachea may occur during the blunt intrathoracic mobilization of the oesophagus. When the damage is significant, the defect

Table 12.2 *Bleeding problems and their solution*

Source of bleeding	Solution
Neck	
External carotid artery	Ligation
Internal carotid	Repair or replace with graft
Internal jugular vein	
Upper end	Ligation following retract digastric muscle ± mandibulotomy
Lower end	Ligation following splitting sternum repair
Thorax	
Oesophageal vessels	Conservative
Azygos vein	Thoracotomy repair

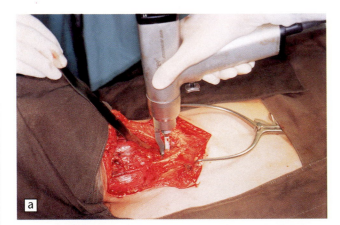

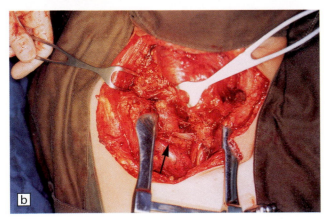

Figure 12.4 (a) The sternum is split in the midline with a sternotome. (b) The sternum is retracted to allow control of the innominate vein (arrow) in the anterior mediastinum.

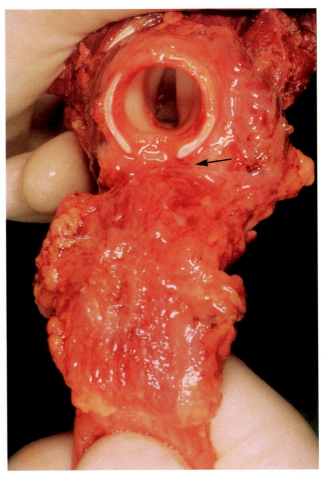

Figure 12.5 Resected specimen showing that the tumour in the cervical oesophagus is closely adherent to the posterior tracheal wall (arrow).

in the posterior tracheal wall may be palpable. More frequently, the injury may be limited and the first sign of any such problem may be the inability of the anaesthetist to keep the patient adequately ventilated. The anaesthetic gas may be leaking through the injured posterior tracheal wall into the mediastinum. Once this is recognized, immediate remedial measures are necessary to restore ventilation. Thoracotomy is mandatory to identify the location and extent of tracheal injury. The patient may be left in the supine position and the upper midline incision continued to a thoracotomy (Fig. 12.7).

The endotracheal tube should be pushed further inferiorly to bypass the damaged tracheal wall; this usually involves the soft tissue of the posterior wall. Depending on the location of the damage, the endotracheal tube can be guided into one of the main bronchi and the patient can be maintained on one-lung ventilation. The damaged tracheal wall can be repaired directly, or a parietal pleural flap can be used for reconstruction (Fig. 12.8). Mobilization of the stomach through the posterior mediastinum to the neck provides additional support to the repaired posterior tracheal wall [2] (Table 12.3).

Damage of other structures

Pylorus

Pyloromyotomy is usually carried out during preparation of the stomach for transposition to the neck. During the procedure, the mucosa at the pylorus may be damaged and the lumen of the duodenum entered inadvertently; in this situation, the pyloromyotomy should be converted

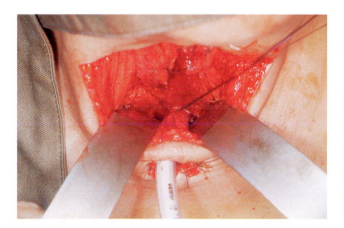

Figure 12.6 The damaged tracheal wall can be repaired from the neck, with the insertion of an endotracheal tube into the terminal tracheostomy to beyond the damaged posterior tracheal wall.

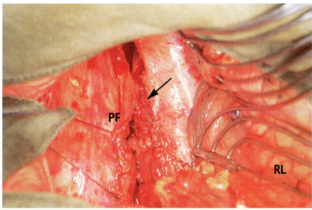

Figure 12.8 Intraoperative photograph through the right thoracotomy. The torn posterior tracheal wall was repaired (arrow) and reinforced with a parietal pleural flap (PF). Note that the right lung (RL) was re-inflated.

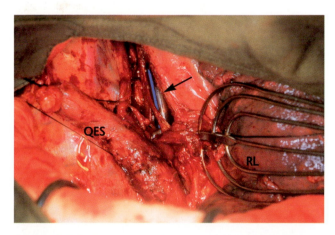

Figure 12.7 Intraoperative photograph through a right thoracotomy. The posterior tracheal wall was damaged during the blunt dissection separating the oesophagus (OES) from the trachea. The endotracheal tube (arrow) is pushed down the left main bronchus to keep the patient ventilated. The right lung (RL) is collapsed and not ventilated.

Table 12.3 *Problems other than bleeding, and their solution*

Problem	Solution
Tracheal wall damage	
High	Repair from neck
Low	Thoracotomy and repair
Pylorus	
During operation	Convert to pyloroplasty
Detected after operation	Roux-en-Y jejunal loop
Spinal accessory nerve (XI)	Direct anastomosis or nerve graft
Phrenic nerve	Direct repair Postoperative chest physiotherapy

into a pyloroplasty. This will eliminate the problem of healing at the pylorus, although it slightly shortens the length of the stomach and affects the final height that the fundus of the stomach may reach.

Spinal accessory nerve

The spinal accessory nerve may be damaged during the neck dissection performed with resection of the primary hypopharyngeal carcinoma. When the nerve is divided without loss of length, the divided nerve ends should be sutured under magnification to allow regeneration. As this is a motor nerve, there is still a chance of recovery. When a segment of nerve is removed because of tumour involvement, a segment of sural nerve may be employed as interposition graft, although the degree of functional recovery under these circumstances is uncertain.

Phrenic nerve

The phrenic nerve may also be damaged during the associated radical neck dissection. As this is also a motor nerve, it should be treated as for the spinal accessory nerve, the divided ends being approximated and sutured under magnification. Injury of the phrenic nerve leads to reduced mobility of the diaphragm and less effective cough efforts; hence sputum retention will develop more readily in the postoperative period. These patients should be given extra attention with regard to breathing and coughing exercises during the convalescent period while the nerve recovers (Table 12.3).

Postoperative problems

Recurrent tumour

The most common and disturbing problem associated with resection of hypopharyngeal carcinoma is the recurrence of tumour. This may occur either locally in the area of the primary resection, near the terminal tracheostomy, or in the cervical lymph nodes as regional recurrence (Table 12.4). Local recurrence is probably related to inadequate resection of the primary tumour, and especially the submucosal tumour extension component

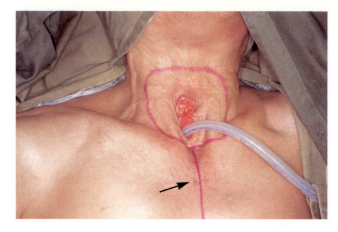

Figure 12.9 Patient with stomal recurrence. The incision marked demonstrates the extent of resection, and the vertical limb of the incision (arrow) allows the exposure of the manubrium part of the sterni for tumour extirpation.

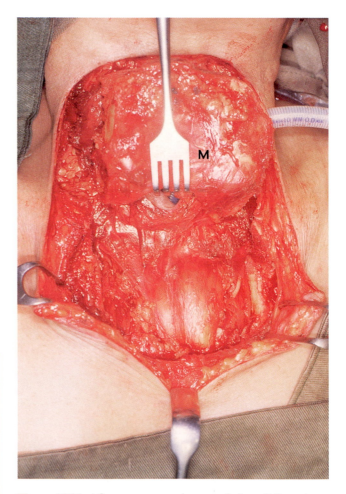

Figure 12.10 After osteotomy, the manubrium (M) can be turned upwards to expose tissue in the anterior mediastinum. The soft tissue and the lymph nodes can be removed under direct vision to ensure clearance.

Table 12.4 *Management of recurrent tumour*

Problem	Solution
Local recurrence	
Tracheal stomal	Resection and mediastinal tracheostomy
Pharyngeal	Resection ± oesophagectomy and reconstruction
Region recurrence	Radical neck dissection

which is common in hypopharyngeal carcinoma. The residual microscopic recurrent tumour in the paratracheal lymph nodes may present as tracheostomal recurrence, while those in the cervical lymph nodes may present as regional metastases.

Local recurrence

When local recurrence in the field of the primary resection is limited, further resection and reconstruction may still provide salvage. However, this is unusual as on detection most local recurrence usually exhibits extensive local infiltration and curative therapy is not possible.

For the recurrence that occurs around the terminal tracheostomy, further curative resection is more likely if such recurrence involves only the upper part of the tracheostomy [3]. Curative resection will include the removal of skin around the recurrence, the terminal segments of the trachea and the manubrium sterni (Fig. 12.9). Removing the manubrium exposes the anterior mediastinum, and soft tissue in the region can be removed together with the recurrence (Fig. 12.10). This manoeuvre also allows the shortened tracheal end to be brought out at a lower position, the mediastinal tracheostomy (Figs 12.11, 12.12).

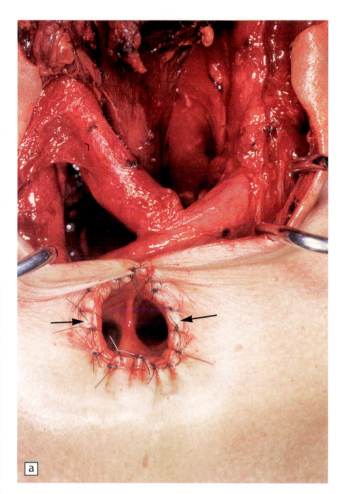

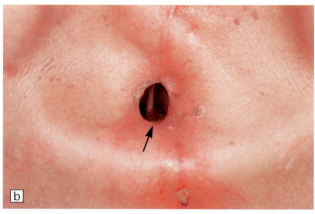

Figure 12.12 (a) Mediastinal terminal tracheostomy constructed in a thin patient. The tracheal stump was short, and the carina is visible through the terminal tracheostome with the opening of the two main bronchi (arrows). (b) The same patient in the postoperative period, showing the terminal tracheostome and the visible carina (arrow).

Figure 12.11 After anterior mediastinal dissection, the great vessels can be identified. The trachea (arrow) can also be divided at a lower level for mediastinal tracheostomy.

As the deep surface of the local recurrence is usually situated close to the cervical oesophagus, the surgical salvage frequently removes the whole oesophagus. Under these circumstances, the stomach must be transposed to the neck for reconstruction. When the skin overlying the manubrium is removed with the bone because of tumour involvement, then the defect can be reconstructed with the pectoralis major myocutaneous flap (Fig. 12.13). Post-operative adjuvant radiotherapy should be given to these patients if the region has not been irradiated previously (Fig. 12.14).

Regional recurrence

Recurrence in the cervical lymph nodes should be treated with radical neck dissection, removing all the lymph nodes and the associated soft tissue. As once metastatic tumour is present in the lymph nodes, the prognosis of the patient is much reduced, every effort should be made to remove all possible sites of tumour seeding. Radical neck dissection is the minimal resection that should be carried out in order to ensure tumour extirpation.

On occasion, when a recurrent lymph node infiltrates the carotid artery, resection of the carotid artery offers salvage in only a small number of patients. The indication for carotid artery resection is that the recurrence is localized, with no other sites of metastasis, and that the resection is a curative one with removal of the segment of carotid artery. Few patients satisfy these criteria and benefit from the resection. The resected segment of carotid artery may be reconstructed with a segment of saphenous vein (Fig. 12.15).

Chylous fistula

When lymphatic output following radical neck dissection reaches a significant amount, then it may pose a problem and contribute to a prolonged period of convalescence.

It is more appropriate if the lymphatic duct can be identified at the primary operation, and ligated. This is

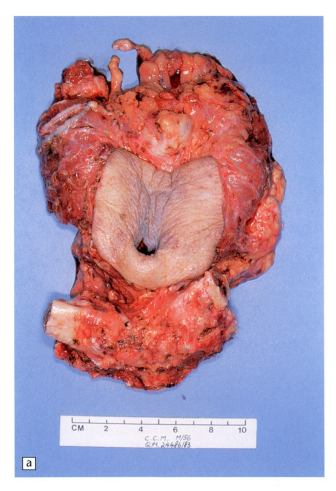

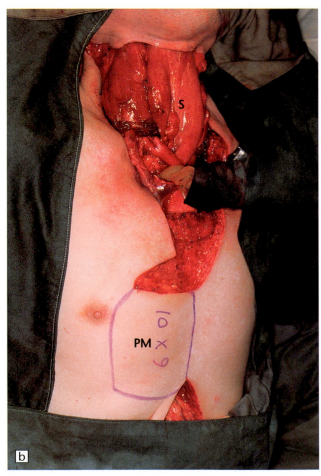

Figure 12.13 (a) The manubrium sterni and the soft tissue in the neck were removed *en bloc* to achieve tumour clearance. (b) The stomach (S) was mobilized to the neck to restore the alimentary tract and the pectoralis major myocutaneous flap (PM) was used to re-surface the neck skin defect.

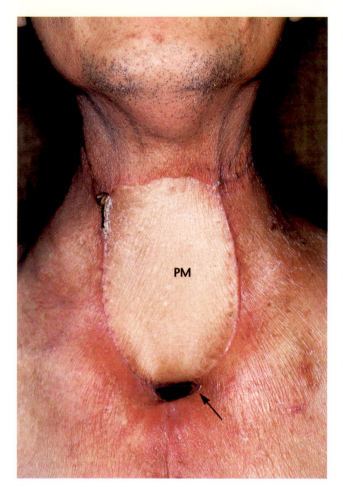

Figure 12.14 Postoperative photograph showing the mediastinal terminal tracheostome (arrow) and the skin island of the pectoralis major myocutaneous flap (PM).

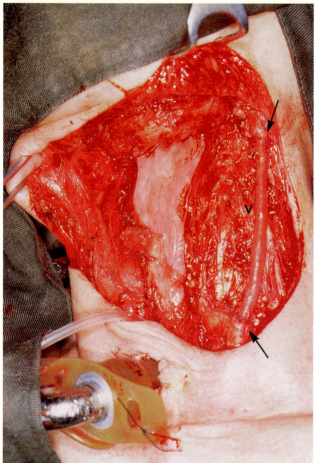

Figure 12.15 Intraoperative photograph showing the replacement of a resected internal carotid artery by a saphenous vein graft (V). The upper and lower vascular anastomoses are shown (arrows).

especially the case when surgery is carried out on the left side of the neck. The left thoracic duct arising from the mediastinum and curving laterally to empty into the junction of the internal jugular vein and the subclavian vein should be identified and ligated at the time of the operation (Fig. 12.16). During surgery, small leakages of lymph may be identified by increasing the intrathoracic pressure. The anaesthetist can contribute in this respect by manually ventilating the patient for 1 minute. With this increased intrathoracic pressure, any significant leakage of lymph in the neck may be identified and secured.

Established small lymphatic leaks normally subside with local pressure dressing. During this time, an elementary diet (medium chain triglyceride) can be administered, or intravenous feeding given. For significant leaks, exploration of the neck with ligation of the lymphatic duct is indicated (Box 12.1).

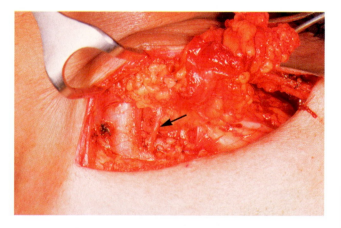

Figure 12.16 Intraoperative photograph showing the left thoracic duct (arrow) during neck dissection. The duct and its branches should be secured before closure of the neck skin to avoid postoperative chylous fistula.

Reconstruction-related problems

Intraoperative problems

Tension at anastomosis

As described in previous chapters, the nature of the tissue employed for reconstruction of the hypopharynx depends on the resultant defect after resection of the primary tumour.

Essentially, patched myocutaneous flap, free jejunal graft and stomach are the tissues frequently used. When the myocutaneous flap is used, the size of the skin island used for reconstruction of the partial hypopharyngeal defect should be designed to avoid any tension along the suture line. The muscle bulk over the vascular pedicle of the pectoralis major myocutaneous flap should be removed so as to avoid any traction when it is placed over the clavicle [4] (Fig. 12.17).

When the free jejunal graft is used for reconstruction of circumferential pharyngeal defects, an adequate length of jejunum should be used. As abundant jejunal tissue is available, then the adequate length of jejunum should be transferred to the neck in order to avoid any tension at the visceral anastomosis. As the diameter of the oropharynx is larger than that of the jejunum, incision over the anti-mesenteric border of the jejunum is necessary to increase the circumference for anastomosis. This will result in some loss of jejunal length, and this should be included in the estimation of the length of the jejunal segment. The jejunum also shrinks once it is manipulated or when the vascular clamps are applied; thus, all measurements should be made before dissection and manipulation of the bowel. This ensures accurate judgement in transferring the appropriate length of jejunum to the neck for reconstruction.

When the stomach is used for reconstruction, it is usually transposed to the neck through the posterior mediastinum (in contrast to the retrosternal or subcutaneous route), as this has been recognized as the shortest route [5]. In addition, the ways to reduce tension at

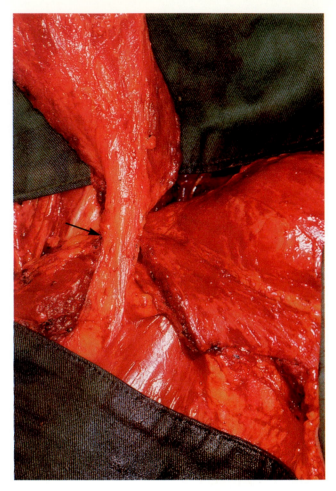

Figure 12.17 Intraoperative photograph showing the vascular pedicle of the pectoralis major myocutaneous flap lying directly over the clavicle (arrow). The sternocostal portion of the pectoralis major muscle was divided.

the pharyngogastric anastomosis involve either mobilizing the pharynx or increasing the length of the stomach.

First, mobilization of the duodenum should be down to its third part; the duodenum lying over the anterior surface of the inferior vena cava should be lifted in total, and freed. The limitation of upward displacement of the duodenum is the entrance of the common bile duct. Second, closure of the cardia should be carried out while at the same time stretching the nearby gastric wall to prevent any 'concertina effect'. This is best achieved when the closure is performed with continuous locking stitches, or alternatively a linear stapler is used to close the cardia (Fig. 12.18). Third, the posterior pharyngeal wall can be mobilized by blunt dissection. The soft tissue plane between the posterior pharyngeal wall and the prevertebral fascia is separated, extending from the oropharynx up to the nasopharynx. This manoeuvre allows the posterior wall of the pharynx to move down by about 1 cm (Fig. 12.19).

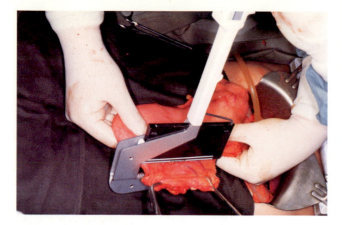

Figure 12.18 The cardia of the stomach is closed with a linear staple while the gastric wall is gently stretched. This reduces the concertina effect following closure of the cardia, and thus prevents shortening of the stomach.

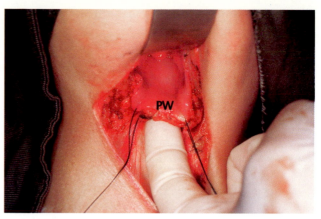

Figure 12.19 The posterior pharyngeal wall (PW) is lifted and, with blunt dissection, is separated from the prevertebral muscle. This manoeuvre will lower the posterior pharyngeal wall suture line.

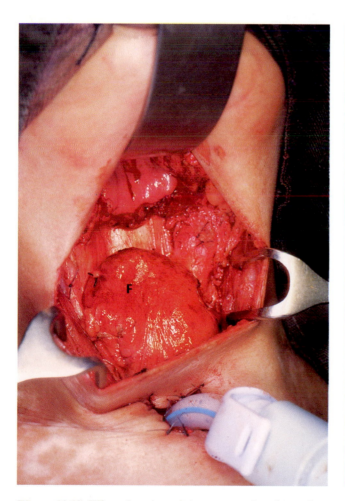

Figure 12.20 When the stomach is transposed to the neck through the posterior mediastinum, the highest point is the dome-shaped fundus (F).

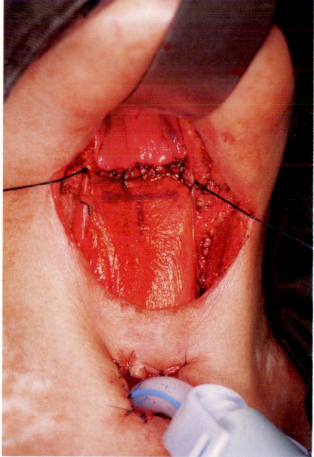

Figure 12.21 The incision over the anterior wall of the stomach is in a 'T'-shaped fashion rather than a linear one. This contributes to better size matching between the pharynx and the stomach.

The lateral part of the pharyngogastric anastomosis normally has the greatest tension. This is because the lateral wall of the pharynx is fixed by the tonsils and cannot move down, while the fundus of the stomach when approaching the neck is in the shape of a dome (Fig. 12.20). The lateral aspect of the stomach must be pulled up for anastomosis. In order to reduce the tension at the suture line, the incision over the stomach should be made in a 'T' fashion rather than a linear one (Fig. 12.21). With this 'gastrotomy' the anterior wall of the stomach can be 'borrowed' to move upward laterally and provide tissue for the lateral aspect (Fig. 12.22). The vertical limb of the 'T' incision, however, lowers the opening over the anterior wall of the stomach. This usually does not matter, as anteriorly the base of the tongue can always descend to reach a lower level to meet the anterior wall of the stomach for the anastomosis. In these ways, the tension at the pharyngogastric anastomosis can be reduced (Box 12.2).

Postoperative problems

During the early postoperative period, the viability of tissue used for reconstruction should be monitored. It is

> **Box 12.2** *Measures to reduce tension at anastomosis*
>
> - Provide adequate tissue for reconstruction
> - Mobilize pharyngeal wall up to the nasopharynx
> - Prevent shortening of stomach on closing the cardia
> - Move anterior wall of stomach laterally for pharyngogastric anastomosis (T-incision on anterior wall of stomach)

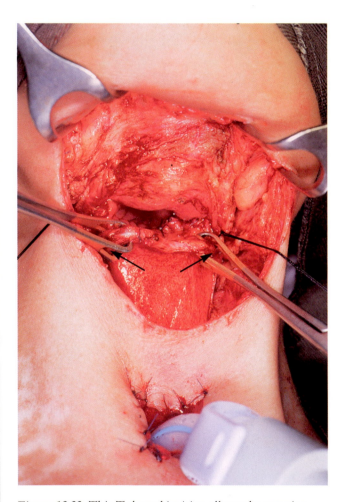

Figure 12.22 This T-shaped incision allows the anterior wall of the stomach to move up laterally to reduce tension over the lateral aspect of the pharyngogastric anastomosis (arrows).

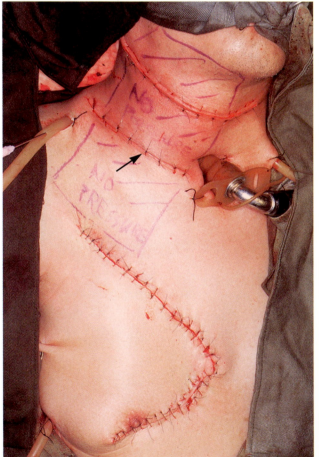

Figure 12.23 The whole area of neck skin over the pectoralis major myocutaneous muscle should be exposed to avoid any inadvertent compression, jeopardizing the blood supply. The pulsation of the vascular pedicle can be felt directly over the clavicle (arrow).

difficult to observe viability of the skin island of the pectoralis major myocutaneous flap because of its location; that of the pectoralis major muscle can usually be monitored by palpation of the pulsation of its feeder artery over the clavicle. Any compression over its pedicle or over the muscle bulk should be avoided. Indeed, the area of skin in the neck overlying the pectoralis major muscle should be exposed to avoid any inadvertent compression (Fig. 12.23).

Loss of jejunal graft

When a segment of jejunum is transferred for pharyngeal reconstruction, its viability should be ensured on completion of the vascular anastomosis, under magnification. The viability of the jejunum is monitored by flexible endoscopic examination. As the jejunal graft can tolerate only a short period of ischaemia, it is difficult to intervene in time to salvage the ischaemic jejunal graft. More frequently, when reduced blood supply is detected, the jejunal graft is completely lost.

The failed jejunal segment should be removed as soon as it is detected and the region cleaned to avoid further infection and sepsis. As the neck region is usually contaminated with saliva and other pathogens, immediate reconstruction should be avoided. Adequate coverage of the region should be carried out with minimal dissection and the patient supported with adequate nutritional care. When the patient recovers from this episode, then a further reconstructive procedure is indicated (Box 12.3).

At the time of removing the non-viable jejunal segment, the region should be irrigated with an ample volume of fluid to reduce contamination. A deltopectoral flap may then be raised to cover the exposed prevertebral fascia and muscle (Fig. 12.24). The upper part of this flap should be sutured to the lower edge of the posterior wall of the oropharynx, while the lower part of the flap is joined with the posterior half of the upper end of the cervical oesophagus. This deltopectoral flap serves to cover the wound area in the neck and forms the posterior wall of the future neopharynx. The anterior wall of the oropharynx is sutured to the edge of the upper neck skin flap to form a pharyngostoma (Fig. 12.25). The anterior

edge of the cervical oesophagus is sutured to the lower neck skin flap to form the cervical oesophagostome (Fig. 12.26).

Enteric feeding is possible with a gastric tube inserted through the cervical oesophagus. The output from the pharyngostoma can be collected into a bag to reduce

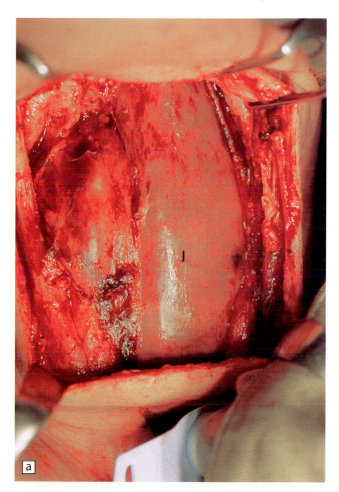

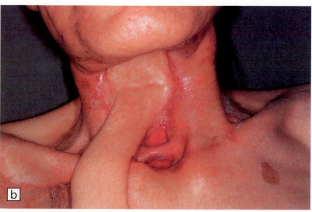

Figure 12.24 (a) A non-viable jejunal graft (J). (b) After removing the jejunal graft, a deltopectoral flap was used to cover the prevertebral fascia. This also acted as the posterior wall of the future neopharynx.

Box 12.3 *Management of lost jejunal free graft*

- Removal of non-viable jejunal graft
- Construction of pharyngostome and oesophagostome
- Deltopectoral flap for reconstruction of posterior pharyngeal wall
- Second-stage reconstruction of anterior pharyngeal wall using a myocutaneous flap

contamination. When all the wounds have healed and the patient has recovered from this episode, then a pectoralis major myocutaneous flap can be raised for reconstruction (Fig. 12.27). The skin island can be used to form the anterior wall of the neopharynx to restore continuity of the alimentary tract reconstituted. A split thickness skin graft can then be applied over the muscle bulk of the pectoralis major myocutaneous flap (Fig. 12.28).

Leakage from pharyngeal reconstruction

Leakage from the reconstructed pharynx may manifest both in the early or late postoperative period. A number of factors may contribute to the leakage of the pharyngeal closure, including previous radiotherapy, the nutritional condition of the patient, and also the technique used to reconstruct the pharynx.

Minor leakage

This usually occurs in the relatively late postoperative period and is detected by a barium swallow. The local clinical condition of the patient governs the management. When the leakage is only shown on radiological examination with no local infection or inflammation, then conservative treatment should be instituted. This includes feeding through a nasogastric tube, thus bypassing the leakage region. A small sinus or fistula usually heals within 2–3 weeks.

When there are signs of infection and local tissue reaction, then the wound close to the leakage site should be opened up to provide a direct drainage. The site of opening of the neck wound should be selected to be away from the terminal tracheostomy. This is to prevent either drainage of saliva or discharge from the fistula from passing down the trachea. Early drainage of

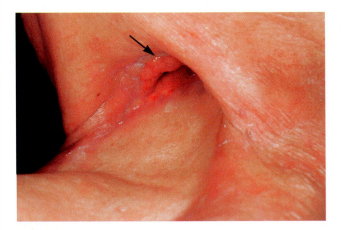

Figure 12.25 The base of the tongue is sutured to the chin skin (arrow), and this forms the pharyngostome.

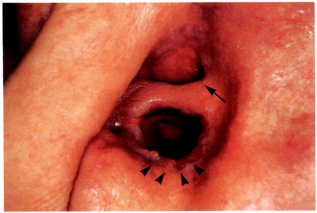

Figure 12.26 The lower edge of the deltopectoral flap was sutured to the posterior part of the cervical oesophageal opening to form a complete oesophagostome (arrow) lying behind the terminal tracheostome (arrowheads).

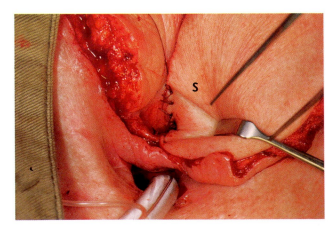

Figure 12.27 A pectoralis major myocutaneous flap is raised at a second stage and its skin island (S) is used to reconstruct the anterior wall of the neopharynx.

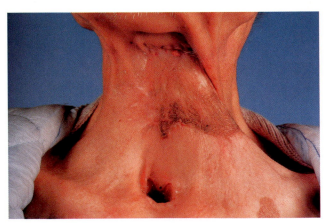

Figure 12.28 Postoperative photograph of the patient in Fig. 12.27, showing the split thickness skin graft over the muscle belly of the pectoralis major myocutaneous flap.

Box 12.4 *Management of leakage following pharyngeal reconstruction*

- Minor leakage: conservative treatment
- Major leakage: exteriorization of leakage and, when inflammation subsides, second-stage reconstruction

suspected leakage is important in order to prevent the accumulation of saliva and infected material in the tissue, as this may lead to more extensive inflammation and necrosis (Box 12.4).

Major leakage

Significant dehiscence of the pharyngeal closure usually manifests in the early postoperative period as wound erythema and oedema. Once this is suspected, the patient should be re-explored and the leakage site identified. The dehiscent wound should be exteriorized by suturing the healthy mucosa to the nearby cutaneous element. The leakage should be converted into a controlled pharyngostoma (Fig. 12.29). In this way, the spread of infection to the surrounding areas (and possible sequelae of tissue necrosis) can be prevented. This modality of treatment should also be applied to those minor leakages that do not respond well to simple drainage.

When the inflammation subsides and the wound has healed, the created pharyngostoma can be reconstructed with a pectoralis major myocutaneous flap (Fig. 12.30).

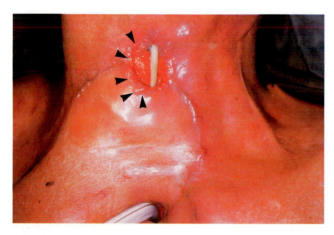

Figure 12.29 Leakage from a pharyngogastric anastomosis is identified and converted into a controlled pharyngostome (arrowheads).

Summary

Understanding the development of intraoperative and postoperative complications will alert the surgeon to take measures to prevent their occurrence. However, on occasion – despite all precautions having been taken – the patient still develops complications that are related either to resection or reconstruction. The early recognition of these complications, associated with their prompt and appropriate management, will reduce the subsequent morbidity among patients.

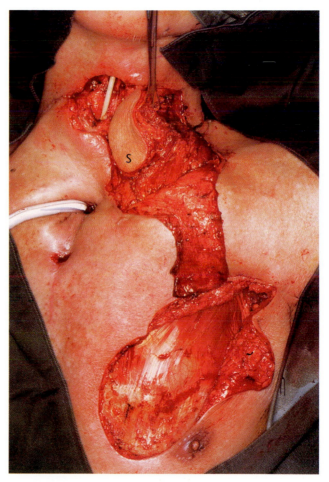

Figure 12.30 The skin island (S) from a pectoralis major myocutaneous flap is used to close the pharyngostome when all the infection and oedema has subsided.

References

1. Wei WI, Lam LK, Yuen PW, J Wong. Current status of pharyngolaryngo-esophagectomy and pharyngogastric anastomosis. *Head Neck* 1998; 20: 240–244.

2. Wei WI, Lam KH, Lau WF *et al*. Salvageable mediastinal problems in pharyngolaryngo-esophagectomy and pharyngogastric anastomosis. *Head Neck Surg* 1988; 10: S60–S68.

3. Sisson GA, Bytell DE, Becker SP. Mediastinal dissection – 1976: indications and newer techniques. *Laryngoscope* 1977; 87: 751–759.

4. Wei WI, Lam KH, Wong J. The true pectoralis major myocutaneous island flap: an anatomical study. *Br J Plast Surg* 1984; 37: 568–573.

5. Ngan SY, Wong J. Lengths of different routes for oesophageal replacement. *J Thorac Cardiovasc Surg* 1986; 91: 790–792.